'Writers write, yes, but *why* tu— anyone could ask. Is it because or because we would otherwis a source of joy or of dread, ar. difficulty that we live for our next page or fear it will kill us; ... of the writers here writing seems to be a process of felicitous discovery, it is perhaps no surprise that this compendium as a whole, too, crackles with the freshness of truths just-now-popping-to-mind. I was astonished by the beauty, candor, and insight of these pieces, every one of which finally helps articulate the ineffable. Marvelous!'

Gish Jen, *author of* Thank You, Mr. Nixon

'In *Driven to Write*, Ellen Pinsky and Michael Slevin have gathered a scribe's tribe—scholars, poets, novelists, songwriters—as diverse in their motives as in their modes of making. To read these essays is to sit around a fire while the wise ones wax. Part observation, part ode, eclectic and electric, this collection is a must have for writers and readers alike.'

John Murillo, *author of* Kontemporary Amerikan Poetry

'A remarkable volume featuring more than 40 writers reflecting on what drives them to write. Personal, poignant, sad, humorous—each testimonial is unique; taken together, they show that writing emanates from deep within a writer's soul. The first collection to explore so intimately the allure of writing, *Driven to Write* is a literary treasure for writers, and for anyone who reads their works.'

Lissa Muscatine, *Politics and Prose Bookstore*

'A fascinating look at the urges and desires of the writing artist, from Louise Glück's belief in a voice more immutable than speech to Carl Phillips' discovery that 'the poem tends to know what we don't yet know,' from Adam Phillips' writing as dreaming to Ha Jin's writing as faith. As Jane Leavy's father once told her, "Writers write." But why? For those of us who ask that question, this book offers so much to learn from and think about.'

Elisa Gabbert, *author of* Any Person Is the Only Self

'"What drives you to write?" I love the simplicity and directness of the question, the complexity and variety of the responses. A single question bringing out a wide range of experiences that can and somehow *must* be expressed through words on a page. Writing is doing, an action. These personal essays, from an impressive gathering of "doers", offer fascinating insights into the impulse behind it.'

Jeffrey Brown, *PBS News Hour*

Driven to Write

In this book of essays, over 40 successful writers in varied fields—poetry, science, the performing and visual arts, psychoanalysis, journalism, literature and more—explore what drives them to write, and to work at their craft.

In contributions arranged under three headings—"Models and Mentors," "Urges and Traumas" and "Evidence and Experiences"—each writer explores their personal understanding of writing as a psychological necessity. In varying ways, these candid, often emotional essays reveal a range of intimate, mysterious and unpredictable purposes and motivations.

Driven to Write provides fresh, practical, and imaginative approaches to literary art for aspiring and established writers alike.

Ellen Pinsky is the author of *Mortal Gifts* (2017), described by one reviewer as "[a] book to be read alongside Freud's Papers on Technique." Her writing about psychoanalysis and her clinical work have been enriched by years of experience as a middle school English teacher.

Michael Slevin is an editor, writer, and psychoanalytic therapist. An expansive curiosity informs his work as a journalist and as a clinician. He co-edited *The Trauma of Racism: Lessons from the Therapeutic Encounter* (2023).

Driven to Write

45 Writers on the Motives and Mysteries of Their Craft

Edited by Ellen Pinsky and Michael Slevin

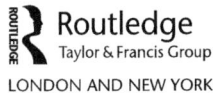
Routledge
Taylor & Francis Group

LONDON AND NEW YORK

Designed cover image: ©Betty Crews

First published 2026
by Routledge
4 Park Square, Milton Park, Abingdon, Oxon OX14 4RN

and by Routledge
605 Third Avenue, New York, NY 10158

Routledge is an imprint of the Taylor & Francis Group, an informa business

© 2026 selection and editorial matter, Ellen Pinsky and
Michael Slevin; individual chapters, the contributors

The right of Ellen Pinsky and Michael Slevin to be identified as the
authors of the editorial material, and of the authors for their individual
chapters, has been asserted in accordance with sections 77 and 78 of the
Copyright, Designs and Patents Act 1988.

All rights reserved. No part of this book may be reprinted or reproduced
or utilised in any form or by any electronic, mechanical, or other means,
now known or hereafter invented, including photocopying and recording,
or in any information storage or retrieval system, without permission in
writing from the publishers.

Trademark notice: Product or corporate names may be trademarks
or registered trademarks, and are used only for identification and
explanation without intent to infringe.

British Library Cataloguing-in-Publication Data
A catalogue record for this book is available from the British Library

ISBN: 978-1-032-85009-2 (hbk)
ISBN: 978-1-032-85011-5 (pbk)
ISBN: 978-1-003-51611-8 (ebk)

DOI: 10.4324/9781003516118

Typeset in Optima
by Apex CoVantage, LLC

The Question
When did you know you wanted to become
A poet? No one believes this question.
No one listens for the answer. It's one
Of those habits of people forced to live
Together on a spinning rock, the pale
Blue dot a wince in the wide attention
The dying light seeks out from ice giants
Dull and firm in the dark, under polite
Lights, midst rows and rows of people who ask
When and why about poetry, of she
Who forgets to ask something that was,
I realize later, part of the poem,
The part where it all comes together, and,
Having come together, finally sings.

Permissions Line UK: Rowan Ricardo Phillips, "The Question" from *Living Weapon*. Copyright © 2021 by Rowan Ricardo Phillips. Reprinted with the permission of Faber and Faber Ltd.

Permissions Line US: "The Question" from LIVING WEAPON by Rowan Ricardo Phillips. Copyright © 2018 by Rowan Ricardo Phillips. Reprinted by permission of Farrar, Straus and Giroux. All rights reserved.

Contents

**2
Urges and Traumas**

Author Biographies

Anne Adelman is a clinical psychologist and Teaching and Training Analyst at the Washington Baltimore Center for Psychoanalysis, and a recipient of that institute's award for excellence in teaching in 2019. She is also a Teaching Analyst at the Contemporary Freudian Society. She has published several articles and is the co-author and editor of four books: *When The Garden Isn't Eden: More Psychoanalytic Stories from Life,* with Kerry Malawista and Linda Kanefield; *Analytic Reflections on Parenting Teens and Young Adults: Changing Patterns of Modern Love, Loss and Longing; The Therapist in Mourning: From the Faraway Nearby; Wearing my Tutu to Analysis and Other Stories.* As the co-editor of the *Journal of the American Psychoanalytic Association* Review of Books, she launched a feature column called "Why I Write," inviting analysts to reflect on the experience of writing. She is a co-chair of the New Directions in Writing Program and maintains a private practice in Chevy Chase, Maryland.

Peg Boyers is Executive Editor of the humanities quarterly *Salmagundi* and author of four books of poems: *Hard Bread, Honey With Tobacco, To Forget Venice* and *The Album.* She currently teaches poetry workshops at Skidmore College and at the New York State Summer Writers Institute.

Robert Boyers is the author of a dozen books, editor of a dozen others, founder and Editor in Chief of the quarterly *Salmagundi,* Director of the New York State Summer Writers Institute and professor of English at Skidmore College. His most recent books are *The Tyranny of Virtue: Identity, The Academy & The Hunt for Political Heresies* (2019), *The Fate of Ideas* (2015) and *Maestros & Monsters: Days & Nights with Susan Sontag & George Steiner* (2023).

Nancy J. Chodorow is a psychoanalyst and professor of sociology emerita, University of California, Berkeley, where she was a founding member of the Gender and Women's Studies Department and the

University of California Interdisciplinary Psychoanalytic Consortium. She is faculty at Harvard Medical School/Cambridge Health Alliance, the Boston Psychoanalytic Society and Institute, and the San Francisco Center for Psychoanalysis. Her first book, *The Reproduction of Mothering*, received the Jessie Bernard Award and was recently honored in Bueskens, ed., *Nancy Chodorow and The Reproduction of Mothering: 40 Years On*. Other books include *Feminism and Psychoanalytic Theory*; *Femininities, Masculinities, Sexualities: Freud and Beyond*; *The Power of Feelings: Personal Meaning in Psychoanalysis, Gender and Culture* (Bryce Boyer Award); *Individualizing Gender and Sexuality: Theory and Practice*; and *The Psychoanalytic Ear and The Sociological Eye: Toward an American Independent Tradition*. Chodorow's writings helped to create feminist theory and psychoanalytic feminism, and brought together psychoanalysis and the social sciences.

Patricia Churchland originated neurophilosophy: approaching philosophical problems in light of insights from contemporary neuroscience. Her 1986 book *Neurophilosophy* was the first major statement of this program, and her book *Touching a Nerve* (2013) was intended for a very broad audience. Her 1992 book *The Computational Brain* (co-authored with Terrence Sejnowski) is a central and influential statement of the foundations of computational neuroscience. She brought insights from neuroscience to questions in ethics and moral philosophy in her books *Braintrust* (2011) and *Conscience* (2019). Her election to the American Academy of Arts and Sciences is particularly apt, both because neurophilosophy is the major emerging field within philosophy and because women are a strongly underrepresented group. She was a MacArthur Fellow (1991) and a recipient of the Rossi Prize in neuroscience (2008). An extended interview can be found on The Science Network (www.tsn.org) and on Philosophy Bites.

Rachel Dillon is a writer, editor and educator from Massachusetts. A former high school English teacher in NYC public schools, she serves as Managing Editor for *Ploughshares* literary journal. Dillon was a recipient of the inaugural Susan Kamil Scholarship for Emerging Writers from the BINC Foundation and has also received support from the Bread Loaf Environmental Writers' Conference, The Kenyon Review Writers Workshop and the Robert Pinsky Global Fellowship. She was a finalist for the 2023 Stephen Dunn Prize, the 2023 Academy of American Poets University Prize and the 2024 Manchester Cathedral Poetry Competition. She is currently writing her first full-length book of poems.

Rita Dove, winner of the 1987 Pulitzer Prize in poetry and U.S. Poet Laureate from 1993 to 1995, received the National Humanities Medal from President Clinton in 1996 and the National Medal of Arts from President Obama in 2011. Among her latest honors are the 2019 Wallace Stevens Award, a 2022 Ruth Lilly Poetry Prize and the 2023 honorary National Book Award. Her most recent books include *Collected Poems 1974–2004* and *Playlist for the Apocalypse*. Her drama *The Darker Face of the Earth* was staged at the Kennedy Center in Washington and the National Theatre in London, and her song cycles with composers John Williams, Tania Leon, Richard Danielpour and others were performed at Tanglewood, New York's Lincoln Center, and the Kennedy Center. She teaches creative writing at the University of Virginia and, since 2023, serves as vice president for literature of the American Academy of Arts & Letters.

Nazila Fathi is the author of *The Lonely War: One Woman's Account of the Struggle for Modern Iran* (*The Guardian*, *Vogue* and Foreign Policy Association named it the best non-fiction of 2014). She reported out of Iran for the New York Times for nearly two decades until 2009, when government threats forced her to leave the country. She translated *History and Documentation of Human Rights in Iran*, by Nobel Peace Prize Laureate Shirin Ebadi, into English. Fathi has also written five children's books. She lives in Bethesda, MD.

Louise Glück, who died in 2023, was the author of two collections of essays and thirteen books of poems. Her many awards include the Nobel Prize in Literature, the National Humanities Medal, the Pulitzer Prize for *The Wild Iris*, the National Book Award for *Faithful and Virtuous Night*, the National Book Critics Circle Award for *The Triumph of Achilles*, the Bollingen Prize for Poetry, the Los Angeles Times Book Prize for *Poems 1962–2012* and the Wallace Stevens Award from the Academy of American Poets.

Among the best-known of **Stephen Greenblatt**'s fourteen books are *Will in the World: How Shakespeare Became Shakespeare*; *The Swerve: How the World Became Modern*; *The Rise and Fall of Adam and Eve*; and *Tyrant: Shakespeare on Politics*. His awards include the Pulitzer Prize, the National Book Award, the Holberg Prize, the Guggenheim Fellowship (twice) and the James Russell Lowell Prize (twice). He is General Editor of The Norton Anthology of English Literature and The Norton Shakespeare. He is a member of the American Academy of Arts and Letters, the American Academy of Arts and Sciences, the American Philosophical Society, Italy's Academia degli Arcadi, the British Academy and Germany's Orden Pour le Mérite für Wissenschaften und Künste. Greenblatt lives in Cambridge, Massachusetts and teaches at Harvard.

Bill Griffith is the creator of the long-running daily comic strip *Zippy the Pinhead*. He began his career in Underground Comix in 1970. Since 2014, he has published three graphic novels. The most recent, *Three Rocks*, is a biography of *Nancy* comics creator Ernie Bushmiller. He is currently at work on a fourth graphic novel and lives quietly, deep in the Connecticut woods.

Forrest Hamer is an Oakland psychologist and psychoanalyst who teaches at the San Francisco Center for Psychoanalysis and the Northern California Society for Psychoanalytic Psychology. The author of three books of poetry—*Call and Response* (Alice James, 1995), winner of Beatrice Hawley Award; *Middle Ear* (Roundhouse, 2000), winner of the Northern California Book Award; and *Rift* (Four Way Books, 2007)—he has also authored articles on race and psychoanalysis, one of which, "Guards at the Gate: Race, Resistance and Psychic Reality," won the 2000 Affiliate Council Prize from the American Psychoanalytic Association. He is a former lecturer at the University of California, Berkeley, in psychology and in the School of Social Welfare.

Julius W. Hobson, Jr. has over fifty years of experience dealing with the Congress and Federal departments and agencies. As Senior Policy Advisor at Polsinelli, he advises and lobbies on a number of issues. Mr. Hobson previously served as lobbyist and Director of Congressional Affairs, American Medical Association. Prior to joining the AMA, Mr. Hobson served on the staff of Senator Charles Robb [D-VA]. He previously served as Congressional and Executive Branch liaison for the District of Columbia Government, Executive Office of the Mayor. Mr. Hobson was Chief of Staff to a Member of Congress and Staff Director of a House Subcommittee. He also handled Congressional and Federal Affairs for Howard University. Mr. Hobson served a four-year term as an elected member of the D.C. Board of Education. Mr. Hobson is Adjunct Professor, Graduate School of Political Management, George Washington University, where he teaches lobbying and legislative writing and research.

Ha Jin was born in 1956 in Jin County, Liaoning Province. At age fourteen, he served in the PLA (People's Liberation Army), staying on the Sino-Soviet border in Hunchun, Jilin. He left mainland China for America in 1985 to do graduate work at Brandeis University, earning his PhD in English and American literature in 1993. Since the early 1990s, he has been writing in both English and Chinese. He is the author of more than twenty books. In English he has published nine novels, four short story collections, four volumes of poetry, a book of essays and a biography of Li Bai. His awards include the National Book Award, two PEN/Faulkner Awards, the PEN/Hemingway Award, the Flannery O'Connor Award for Short Fiction and the Asian American Literary Award. Currently he teaches fiction writing and migrant literature at Boston University, where he is William Fairfield Warren Distinguished Professor. He lives outside Boston with his family.

Judy L. Kantrowitz's active love of reading fiction stirred her longings to write fiction herself, but she found her abilities were far better suited to being a psychoanalyst. Exploring character and conflict with people, not just writing about it, was more compatible with her social nature; it also offered her the opportunity to train, supervise and teach future psychoanalysts at the Boston Psychoanalytic Institute. Over time, her work with patients led her back to writing as she found herself discovering how both she and her patients learned about themselves through working together in a psychoanalytic process. Kantrowitz is the author of four books, most recently *The Role of Patient-Analyst Match in the Process and Outcome of Psychoanalysis*. She has served on the editorial board of the *Journal of the American Psychoanalytic Association*. In 2020, she won their prize for her paper "A Psychoanalytic Memoir." She is in private practice in Brookline, MA.

Joseph Leo Koerner is Chair of the Department of History of Art and Architecture and Senior Fellow of the Society of Fellows, Harvard University. His latest book, *Art in a State of Siege*, explores works by Hieronymus Bosch, Max Beckmann and William Kentridge created and received in dangerous times. He has written and presented arts documentaries for the BBC, and wrote, produced and directed the feature film *The Burning Child*.

Jane Leavy is the author of the national bestsellers *The Big Fella: Babe Ruth and the World He Created*; *The Last Boy: Mickey Mantle and the End of America's Childhood; Sandy Koufax: A Lefty's Legacy*; and the comic novel *Squeeze Play*, which *Entertainment Weekly* called "the best novel ever written about baseball." She was a staff writer at *The Washington Post* from 1979 to 1988, first for the Sports section, then for Style. Her work has been anthologized in many collections, including *The Good Book: Writers Reflect on Favorite Bible Passages; Jewish Jocks: An Unorthodox Hall of Fame; Best Sportswriting; Coach: 25 Writers Reflect on People Who Made a Difference*; and *Child of Mine: Essays on Becoming a Mother*. She has two adult children, Nick and Emma Isakoff. She lives in Washington, D.C., and Truro, Massachusetts.

Robert Jay Lifton is a psychiatrist and author whose subject has been holocaust, mass violence, and renewal in the 20th and 21st centuries. His books include *Death in Life: Survivors of Hiroshima* (winner of a National Book Award); *The Nazi Doctors: Medical Killing and the Psychology of Genocide* (winner of a Los Angeles Times Book Prize); *Home from the War: Learning from Vietnam Veterans* (nominated for a National Book Award); *Thought Reform and the Psychology of Totalism: A Study of "Brainwashing" in China*; and *Witness to an Extreme Century: A Memoir*. His most recent books are *Losing Reality: On Cults, Cultism, and the Mindset of Political and Religious Zealotry* and *Surviving our Catastrophes: Resilience and Renewal from Hiroshima to the Covid-19 Pandemic*. Dr. Lifton is currently Lecturer in Psychiatry at Columbia University and Distinguished Professor Emeritus of Psychiatry and Psychology at the City University of New York.

A former senior speechwriter for President Barack Obama, **David Litt** is the *New York Times* bestselling author of *Thanks, Obama: My Hopey Changey White House Years* and *Democracy in One Book or Less*. He has written for *The New York Times*, *The Atlantic,* the *Washington Post*, *The Los Angeles Times, The Boston Globe* and *Cosmo*, among others. He also continues to write speeches for leading political figures, philanthropists, celebrities and CEOs. Described as the "comic muse for the president" for his work on the White House Correspondents' Dinner monologues, he was also the head writer/producer of Funny or Die, D.C., and has written TV pilots for Comedy Central, ABC and NBC.

Phillip Lopate is a central figure in the revival of the American essay, both through his ubiquitous edited anthology, *Art of the Personal Essay*, and his own essay collections, *Bachelorhood, Against Joie de Vivre, Portrait of My Body, Portrait Inside My Head* and *A Year and a Day*. He is author of the book-length nonfiction works *Being With Children, Waterfront, Notes on Sontag, Rudy Burckhardt: Photographer* and *A Mother's Tale*. Additionally, he has written books of fiction (*Confessions of Summer, The Rug Merchant, Two Marriages*), poetry (*At the End of the Day*) and film criticism (*Totally Tenderly Tragically, My Affair With Art House Cinema*). Finally, he has edited other anthologies (*Writing New York* and *American Movie Critics*) and has recently completed a three-volume historical anthology of the American essay.

Kerry Malawista, PhD, writer, training and supervising psychoanalyst, co-chair of New *Directions in Writing* and founder of *The Things They Carry Project*, offering virtual writing workshops for groups in need of healing. She is the associate editor of the new creative nonfiction section of *The Journal of the American Psychoanalytic*. Her essays have appeared nationally, including in the *New York Times*, the *Washington Post*, the *Baltimore Sun*, the *Boston Globe* and *Delmarva Review*, which nominated her for a Pushcart Prize. She is coauthor of *When the Garden Isn't Eden* (2022), *Wearing my Tutu to Analysis and Other Stories* (2011), and co-editor of *The Therapist in Mourning: From the Faraway Nearby* (2013), *Who's Behind the Couch* (2017) and editor of *The Things They Wrote: A Writing Healing Project*. Her novel *Meet the Moon* was released in 2022.

Marilyn Martin, M.D., MPH is a psychiatrist and psychoanalyst. Dr. Martin has served in various public health roles, including Medical Director of Baltimore County's Bureau of Mental Health to Medical Director of Maryland's Administrative Services agency. She is currently in private practice in Towson and consults with a community mental health center in Baltimore City. She is a national speaker and author of *Saving Our Last Nerve: The Black Woman's Path to Mental Health*. She serves as a teaching analyst with the Washington-Baltimore Institute for Psychoanalysis and is also a member of the National Association of Black Storytellers.

Jean McGarry is Elliot Coleman Professor in The Writing Seminars (emeritus) at Johns Hopkins University. She has published ten works of fiction; the most recent are *Blue Boy* and *No Harm Done*.

Louis Menand is Anne T. and Robert M. Professor of English and Lee Simpkins Family Professor of Arts and Sciences at Harvard. He has been an editor at *The New Republic* (1986–1987), *The New Yorker* (1993–1994) and *The New York Review of Books* (1994–2001). He began writing for *The New Yorker* in 1991 and has been a staff writer since 2001. He is the author of five books, including *The Metaphysical Club*, which won the Pulitzer Prize in History in 2002.

Sigrid Nunez has published nine novels, including *A Feather on the Breath of God*, *The Friend*, *What Are You Going Through* and, most recently, *The Vulnerables*. She is also the author of *Sempre Susan: A Memoir of Susan Sontag*. *The Friend*, a *New York Times* bestseller, won the 2018 National Book Award and was a finalist for the 2020 International Dublin Literary Award. Nunez's other honors include a Whiting Award, a Berlin Prize Fellowship, the Rome Prize in Literature and a Guggenheim Fellowship. Her work has been translated into more than thirty languages.

Thomas H. Ogden, M.D. is the author of thirteen books on the theory and practice of psychoanalysis as well as literary criticism, most recently *Coming to Life in the Consulting Room*, *Reclaiming Unlived Life*; *Creative Readings: Essays on Seminal Analytic Works*; and *Rediscovering*

Psychoanalysis. He has published three novels, *The Parts Left Out, The Hands of Gravity and Chance* and *This Will Do.* His work has been published in more than twenty-five languages. He has received the Sigourney Award for his contributions to psychoanalysis. He practices and teaches psychoanalysis and creative writing in San Francisco and Sonoma, California.

Orlando Patterson is a professor of sociology at Harvard. He is interested in the comparative study of slavery and freedom, ethno-racial inequality and national development in the Caribbean, especially Jamaica. His non-fiction books include *Slavery and Social Death*; *Freedom in the Making of Western Culture,* which won the 1991 National Book Award for Non-Fiction; and *The Confounding Island: Jamaica and the Post-Colonial Predicament,* which won the 2020 AAP Prose Award for Media and Cultural Studies. He has also published three novels. He has advised two Jamaican Prime Ministers and two U.S. Presidents and has written widely in the press, especially the *New York Times,* where for several weeks he was a guest columnist. He is a member of the American Academy of Arts and Sciences, was a Guggenheim Fellow and co-founded Cultural Survival, an advocacy group for indigenous peoples. In 2016, he won the Anisfield-Wolf Book Award for Lifetime Achievement in Literature; in 2020, he was awarded the Order of Merit by the government of Jamaica; and in 2024 he was awarded the Hegel prize by the City of Strattburg for contribution to the humanities.

Adam Phillips, formerly Principal Child Psychotherapist at Charing Cross Hospital, is a writer and psychoanalyst in London.

Carl Phillips is the author, most recently, of *Scattered Snows, to the North* (Farrar, Straus & Giroux, 2024) and *Then the War: And Selected Poems 2007–2020* (Farrar, Straus & Giroux, 2022), which won the 2023 Pulitzer Prize. Phillips's other honors include the Jackson Poetry Prize, the Kingsley Tufts Poetry Award, the Los Angeles Times Book Award, the Aiken Taylor Award for Modern American Poetry and awards and fellowships from the Guggenheim Foundation, the Academy of American Poets, the American Academy of Arts and Letters and the Library of Congress. Phillips has also written three prose books, most recently *My Trade Is Mystery: Seven Meditations from a Life in Writing* (Yale University Press, 2022). After over thirty years teaching at Washington University in St. Louis, Phillips lives on Cape Cod, Massachusetts.

Rowan Ricardo Phillips is the author of the poetry collections *The Ground, Heaven* and *Living Weapon*; a new book, *Silver,* was recently released from, as with the other titles, Farrar, Straus and Giroux.

Phillips is the recipient of a Whiting Award, a Guggenheim Fellowship, the PEN/Joyce Osterweil Award for Poetry, the Anisfield-Wolf Book Prize, the Nicolás Guillén Outstanding Book Award and the PEN/ESPN Award for Literary Sportswriting. He is a frequent contributor to *The New York Times Magazine* and is the poetry editor of *The New Republic.* He divides his time between New York City and Barcelona.

Ellen Pinsky is the author of *Mortal Gifts: Death and Fallibility in the Psychoanalytic Encounter* (2017). One reviewer called it a "dramatic and beautiful book . . . about psychoanalytic ethics." Another wrote: "This is a book to be read alongside Freud's *Papers on Technique.*" *Mortal Gifts* examines risks and vulnerabilities built into the psychoanalytic situation—an endeavor that purposely courts risk, for a time placing one human being *as if* at the center of another's emotional life. In that power-imbalanced relationship behind closed doors, what, Pinsky asks in *Mortal Gifts,* is the patient's protection from abuse? Ellen Pinsky came to psychoanalysis as a second profession following twenty-five years as a middle school English teacher. She says her experience in the classroom with twelve-year-olds taught her most of what she needed to know to become a creditable clinician.

Robert Pinsky's most recent book of poems is *Proverbs of Limbo.* His PoemJazz album of the same title, with musicians including Laurence Hobgood and Mino Cinélu, is available on Spotify and Apple Music. His autobiography is *Jersey Breaks.* As United States Poet Laureate from 1997 to 2000, he founded the Favorite Poem Project.

Warren Poland, writer and psychoanalyst, is author of the books *Intimacy and Separateness* and *Melting the Darkness* as well as a column in *American Imago.* He was a prior editor of the *Journal of the American Psychoanalytic Association Review of Books* and was also on the editorial board of ten other peer reviewed journals. In 2009, he received the Sigourney Award for Distinguished Contributions to Psychoanalysis.

Joshua Prager is the author of three books, most recently *The Family Roe,* a finalist for the 2022 Pulitzer Prize in general nonfiction. A former senior writer for *The Wall Street Journal,* he received a literature award in 2023 from the American Academy of Arts and Letters. He lives in New Jersey with his wife and two daughters. His website is joshuaprager.com.

Josh Ritter is the author of two novels and eleven albums. Originally from Moscow, Idaho, he now lives in Brooklyn with his partner, novelist Haley Tanner, and two daughters currently impersonating eleven crocodiles. Writing is his favorite thing to do, besides the obvious ones.

Philip Schultz is the author of eight poetry collections, including his most recent, *Luxury,* and the Pulitzer Prize–winning *Failure,* a new memoir, *Comforts of the Abyss,* and *The Wherewithal,* a novel in verse. The founder of The Writers Studio, a private school of creative writing, he is a recipient of The Lamont Prize, a Fulbright Scholarship, the Levinson Prize from Poetry magazine and a National Book Award nomination. He resides in East Hampton, NY with his wife, the sculptor Monica Banks.

Lloyd Schwartz has published five books of poetry and a collection of music reviews and has edited three volumes dedicated to the poetry and prose of Elizabeth Bishop. He is the Frederick S. Troy Professor of English Emeritus at the University of Massachusetts Boston and the longtime arts critic for NPR's Fresh Air and Boston's public radio station WBUR. In 2019 he was appointed poet laureate of Somerville, Massachusetts and continues in that position. Among his honors are the Pulitzer Prize for Criticism, three ASCAP-Deems Taylor Awards for his writing on music, and fellowships from the Guggenheim Foundation, NEA and Academy of American Poets for his poetry. His poems have been selected for the Pushcart Prize, The Best American Poetry and The Best of the Best American Poetry. His most recent collection is *Who's on First? New and Selected Poems* (University of Chicago Press).

Nicole Sealey was born in St. Thomas, U.S. Virgin Islands, and raised in Apopka, Florida. She is the author of *The Ferguson Report: An Erasure* and winner of the 2024 OCM Bocas Prize for Poetry, an excerpt from which was awarded the Forward Prize for Best Single Poem. She is also the author of *Ordinary Beast,* a finalist for the Hurston/ Wright Legacy Award, and *The Animal After Whom Other Animals Are Named,* winner of the Drinking Gourd Chapbook Poetry Prize. Her honors include a 2024–2026 Princeton Arts Fellowship, a Cullman Center Fellowship from the New York Public Library, a Rome Prize in Literature from the American Academy in Rome, a Hodder Fellowship from Princeton University, the Stanley Kunitz Memorial Prize from The American Poetry Review, the Poetry International Prize and fellowships from CantoMundo, Cave Canem, the National Endowment for the Arts and the New York Foundation for the Arts. She teaches in the MFA Writers Workshop in Paris program at New York University.

Grant Shreve is a writer and literary scholar based in Baltimore, Maryland. His work has appeared in a range of academic and popular outlets, including *The Washington Post, The Millions* and *Religion & Politics*. He holds a PhD in American Literature from Johns Hopkins University.

Michael Slevin is a writer and editor on psychoanalytic issues. He co-edited *The Trauma of Racism: Lessons from the Therapeutic Encounter* (2022), and has co-edited and written on race for *The Psychoanalytic Study of the Child*. As editor-in-chief of *The American Psychoanalyst,* he broadened the scope of the magazine to include psychoanalytic insight into culture and social issues. He has been active in bringing psychoanalytic ideas and practice into contexts outside the consulting room, to less privileged communities, and into political decision making. A member of the Washington Baltimore Center for Psychoanalysis, he is in private practice in Baltimore, MD.

Peter Slevin is a contributing writer for *The New Yorker* based in Chicago. He has spent much of his career writing for newspapers, spending seven years in Europe for *The Miami Herald* and a decade on the national staff of *The Washington Post,* where he wrote about foreign policy and later traveled the country with an eye to politics and stories between the coasts. His portrait of Michelle Obama—*Michelle Obama: A Life*—was a finalist for the PEN America biography prize. He is a professor at Northwestern University's Medill School of Journalism.

Beverly J. Stoute, MD, a child, adolescent, and adult psychiatrist and psychoanalyst, is a scholar, clinician, educator, advocate, and leader. She has held leadership positions locally and nationally, most recently serving as Co-Chair of the Holmes Commission on Racial Equality in American Psychoanalysis. A Distinguished Fellow of both the American Psychiatric Association and the American Academy of Child and Adolescent Psychiatry, she serves on the faculties of several psychoanalytic training programs, the Emory University School of Medicine and the Morehouse School of Medicine. She has received multiple awards and honors for her work. Her scholarship, taught at training programs across the United States, has been translated into German, Spanish, and Portuguese and was featured in the Freud Museum archives in London. Dr. Stoute maintains a full-time private practice in Atlanta, GA. Her book, *The Trauma of Racism: Lessons from the Therapeutic Encounter*, co-edited with Michael Slevin, was released by Routledge in 2023.

Peggy Tighe deciphers and interprets complex healthcare matters for very busy people, using the written and spoken word to drive action. She spent her career understanding policy problems faced by provider and patient organizations and influencing federal policy and decision-making on their behalf. Peggy's prior experience with two highly visible national healthcare associations—the American Medical Association and the Health Insurance Association of America—as well as with dozens of national coalitions and individual clients, make her unique in this space. Peggy is former president, "Distinguished Member" and "Lifetime Achievement Award" winner of Women in Government Relations, an organization that advances and empowers women through professional development and mentoring. She was also named "Top Lobbyist" for the National Institute of Lobbying and Ethics in 2020, 2022 and 2023. Peggy's mother once confided, "I think I have a book inside of me." Recognizing her mother's likely discomfort, Peggy writes concisely.

Natasha Trethewey served two terms as the 19th Poet Laureate of the United States. She is the author of five collections of poetry, including *Native Guard*—for which she was awarded the 2007 Pulitzer Prize. She's also the author of *Memorial Drive: A Daughter's Memoir*, an instant *New York Times* bestseller, and, most recently, *The House of Being*, a meditation on writing. A Chancellor of the Academy of American Poets since 2019, Trethewey was awarded the 2020 Rebekah Johnson Bobbitt Prize in Poetry for Lifetime Achievement from the Library of Congress, and in 2022 she was the William B. Hart Poet in Residence at the American Academy in Rome. She is a fellow of the American Academy of Arts and Sciences, the American Academy of Arts and Letters and the American Philosophical Society. At Northwestern University, she is Board of Trustees Professor of English.

Harold Varmus, MD, co-recipient of the 1989 Nobel Prize in Physiology or Medicine for studies of the genetic basis of cancer, joined the Meyer Cancer Center of Weill Cornell Medicine as the Lewis Thomas University Professor of Medicine in 2015. He is also a Senior Associate Member of the New York Genome Center, where he helps to develop programs in cancer genomics, and an adjunct professor at Columbia University. Previously, Dr. Varmus was the Director of the National Cancer Institute for five years, the President of Memorial Sloan-Kettering Cancer Center for ten years, Director of the National Institutes of Health for six years and a faculty member at the University of California medical school in San Francisco for over twenty years. He is a graduate of Amherst College and Harvard University in English literature and of Columbia University in medicine. He is the author of about 400 scientific papers and five books, including a 2009 memoir entitled *The Art and Politics of Science* (Norton).

Foreword

Why do some people feel compelled to write? Forty-five writers from various disciplines—including a sportswriter and a scientist, a Shakespeare scholar and a sociologist, poets, fiction writers and psychoanalysts—answer this question with startling, penetrating responses, as various as life itself.

Many of the essays are, to a surprising degree, confessional. Unaware of each other's takes, it is as though these writers of many different kinds are competing to delve as deeply as possible into the genesis of their scribbling habit. All, regardless of what writing genre they normally practice, are analytical—in a broad sense of that adjective, but also as a word for the Freudian process. Perhaps reflecting that the book's two editors are psychotherapists, many (but not all) of the contributors show the influence of psychoanalytic experience, either as clinicians or analysands: a traditional, endlessly debatable association between creativity and "analysis"—in both senses.

Joy can be the reward for writing—that idea emerges throughout these ruminative, often self-mocking accounts. The language is consistently eloquent, bold, intelligent, polished. Many of the pieces are spectacular.

It would be impossible for any writer (or wannabe writer) to read this book without beginning to form their own answers to the prompt. My first inclination was to reach for the glib reply, "I'm no good at anything else, so by process of elimination I had to become a writer." But that isn't strictly true: I probably could have become a lawyer, an academic dean, even a psychotherapist. So I thought—in the spirit of this book, psychoanalytically—about my need to distance myself from my obstreperous family while putting them into an intelligible framework. There was also my love of literature and, stemming from that love, a desire to emulate my author-heroes—possibly even to join them.

Along with joy, the proud achievement of writing is often haunted by anger, revenge, humiliation and shame, intertwined with a love for the powerful music of language. Many of the respondents, from so many different realms, connect their writing to a parent. Whether father or mother, they reach back to these initial, often inadvertent mentors—gratefully or resentfully or some of each. How might the act of writing involve the original family? Is the habit inextricably tied to memory and to mourning the loss of childhood, with composition a way to recover that lost time?

Is it my imagination, or does it seem that guilt attaches to the very act of writing? Is there guilt in having one's say, and egotistically obliging others to listen? Or betraying the secrets of others? Or is it that writing affords so much solitary pleasure that one can only feel embarrassed indulging in such anti-social activity, and apologetic towards those who don't have opportunities to experience the same relief?

For all that authors occasionally claim to hate writing, they keep doing it, which should tell us something. We know Ralph Ellison complained that writing was like opening up a vein, yet—as Grant Shreve points out in his piece—the author of *Invisible Man* continued to add to his second, unfinished novel, long after he had given up any hope of bringing it to resolution in his lifetime. Whatever its difficulties, writing is surely a way of centering yourself while discovering what might lie in the darkness of the mind, lurking in the unconscious. On your best days, it is also a pathway to delight.

Finally, I think of my own desire to do mischief—not to change the world, just shake up some of its more pious, received opinions. To stumble onto something comic while in the act of writing may be what gives me the most pleasure. Others may have entirely different motivations.

These forty-five participants have begun the conversation, setting the bar high with their provocative accounts: fresh, candid and fun to read. Try it yourself. Let's keep the experiment and the mischief going.

—Phillip Lopate

Editors' Acknowledgments

We editors are grateful to this book's contributors for their candor, imagination, cogency and grace.

Among the many people who have helped us, foremost is our editorial assistant Rachel Dillon, whose expertise and poetic intelligence have improved the book and added to our pleasure in working on it. Much gratitude as well to our agent Mike Mungiello for his belief in the project, his tireless effort and steady guidance.

Editors' Introduction

Ellen Pinsky and Michael Slevin

> "Art is a concrete and personal and rather childish thing after all . . . a game of make-believe, of reproduction, very exciting and delightful to people who have an ear for it or an eye for it."
>
> —Willa Cather, *On Writing*, 1949

Why do people make things? Sandcastles, books, clay pots, paintings, films, businesses, jokes, recipes, poems, songs . . . essays? Each kind of making reflects an effort that is both personal and cultural. The essays in this book embody "essay" as a verb, meaning to try something: to go forth on a defined or not yet defined quest.

What drives a writer on that quest? The motivation for writing, like many powerful desires, can reach so deep that it goes beyond explanation. George Orwell, possibly the most admired of all modern essayists, chooses to conclude his 1946 "Why I Write" on an inglorious, even comical, note:

> I see that I have made it appear as though my motives in writing were wholly public-spirited. I don't want to leave that as the final impression. All writers are vain, selfish, and lazy, and at the very bottom of their motives there lies a mystery. Writing a book is a horrible, exhausting struggle, like a long bout of some painful illness. One would never undertake such a thing if one were not driven on by some demon whom one can neither resist or understand. For all one knows that demon is simply the same instinct that makes a baby squall for attention.

Vanity, illness, irresistible demons, squalling babies—it's quite a picture. Writing is exhausting hard work. (We editors, writing this introduction, can feel much like squalling babies driven by an inexplicable demon.) It's a mystery why anyone does it.

DOI: 10.4324/9781003516118-1

A hundred years ago, Sigmund Freud—another gifted essayist—considered a nursery scene: A grandfather watches how his toddler grandson, who has without fuss let his mother leave the room, repeatedly throws his toy, a wooden spool on a string, over the side of his cot, "fort" ("gone"), then pulling it back, exclaims "da" ("there"), thus managing—symbolizing—an experience of loss and recovery. Like the writer, the child makes something that both expresses his dilemma and provides relief. The boy uses his imagination to give shape, meaning and verbal music to his re-enactment of the loss. With language and play comes comfort. The vocal repetition of disappearance and restoration emphasizes the centrality of language in an individual's development, and in culture. The game, playing "gone," Freud writes, is the child's "great cultural achievement"—a fundamental accomplishment not unlike the sandcastles, jokes and songs on our list.

With quests like those of Cather, Orwell and Freud in mind, we invited writers of many different ages and degrees of eminence across professions and disciplines—including poets, journalists, novelists, therapists, a musician, a lawyer, an art historian, a biochemist, a cartoonist, a Shakespeare scholar, a biographer, a political speechwriter, a music critic. We asked them to write about writing, at the core of that activity: *What, as writers, drives you to write?* To our surprise, most of those we invited accepted the simple invitation: 500 to 2000 words in any genre, with a personal voice addressing the question: *Why do you need to write?* Many of our authors expressed surprise at our invitation and were moved to be included. No one before, it seems, had asked them to reach deeply into themselves with this question. As one author put it, in accepting the invitation: "I am intrigued, and eager to find out what I think."

What, in relation to writing, is shared by so many kinds of writers? As editors we noticed recurring tensions: loss and comfort; shame and relief; pain and pleasure; boredom and curiosity; excitement and revenge; hunger and satisfaction; all part of, or subordinate to, an urge that remains a mystery. We found a narrative thread, sometimes implicit, sometimes explicit: Writing is a form of mourning—something is no longer "here" where it was, but is "here" in the essay. "Fort," "da."

Three kinds of motive, broadly defined, emerged as an organizing three-part structure—a triangle, the strongest of shapes:

Models and Mentors—*Who has inspired me:* my father, my mother, my Russian refugee grandma, my friend, my teacher, a stranger on the street, the therapist, my endlessly playful and forgiving cat Max, the author I love, the painter I admire, the musician who transports me, the basketball player whose grace and spunk inspire me.

Urges and Traumas—*What's inside me:* impulse, my struggles, my knacks, my hopes and fears.

Evidence and Experiences—*What I have experienced:* the world, the society, my homeland, a work of art, reality, the audience, the war, the peace, loss, the election, the natural world.

We mean this loose structure to be suggestive, even ambiguous, rather than rigid. A particular essay might arguably fit more than one of the three categories. Some of the pieces of writing fall closer to one point of the triangle, or somewhere between two points. Some are near the exact center. But all of these essays can be located inside the triangle, and all three points are relevant to each piece.

The rich notion of being "driven," too, is manifold: The inspiration is mysterious, the passions are magnetic, and the stories are effective beyond mere reason, the motives unconscious.

As the word "unconscious" may suggest, both of us are psychotherapists. Most of the writers in the volume don't mention psychotherapy, but the two processes—forming words as a patient or as a writer—are related. Sigmund Freud may be too easily dismissed these days. We think our collection tends to confirm, maybe even redeem, some of his insights.

The act of finding words—"fort," "da"—is an emotional accomplishment: something human beings strive to do in many kinds of ways, and not just by writing. The verbal quest goes way back before the invention of the printing press or the pixel—back to the oral tradition, the epic. One writer here remembers cruising in her father's work truck, singing along to the radio: "[A]s 'Bridge over Troubled Water' played on the radio, I was gripped by the lyrics," she writes.

> My mother was still alive then, so I know that I wasn't yet ten years old. It took my breath away to discover that 'bridge' could mean a friend who helps you get over hard times . . . and I could use my words to connect myself to others.

While much varies across disciplines, each word or sentence of good writing is part of an essential quest for reality. We don't analyze or explain these surprising, unique essays, nor do we offer any utilitarian "how to" for aspiring writers. The writing we admire rises above buzzwords, slogans and bromides. Our title, *Driven to Write*, tries to reach beyond formulas, deeper than mere memoir, by touching a need.

Freud asks, in "Creative Writers and Day-dreaming," why do the writer's fantasies not repel us or leave us cold but instead give us pleasure? His answer: the artist positions us to enjoy our own daydreams "without shame or self-reproach." The child, in play, re-ordering the world. The artist deploying form to play upon the instrument of the mind. The pieces in this volume are offered for that pleasure.

A squalling infant, a toddler's game, an 8-year-old child riding in her father's work truck, singing along to the radio. An adolescent boy, to hide his embarrassing myopia, reads road signs through binoculars. An émigré from mainland China muses on his writing in relation to the quasi-religious single word in the Chinese language for "nation" and "country." A student paralyzed by a road accident watches his index finger bend down: "and I saw in its glorious little jerk communication." An art historian, the son of a painter, describes the "pig lady," fearless and cruel, depicted in his father's painting:

> an old lady way less than five feet tall who used to feed bread rolls to the wild boars . . . this tiny woman stirring up these animals into a feeding frenzy, then clubbing them on the nose if they fought over the bread.

A 98-year-old psychohistorian begins his story "with a walk in Hong Kong in late April of 1954, when I was 28 years old" and narrates the decision that made him a writer. The biographer of Sandy Koufax and Babe Ruth remembers being told "Writers write," and each time she hears the simple words, she writes: "And I know who I am."

1

Models and Mentors

Ellen Pinsky and Michael Slevin

Stephen Greenblatt

Professor, Writer

Trust

Why do I write? Because I do not know what I think until I sit down and put my thoughts on paper. And that isn't quite right, because I don't have my thoughts fully formed in my head and then transcribe them; rather they come into my head and take shape and form only when I sit down to write. I am amazed at people who actually know in advance what they are going to write and who create outlines that they follow in dutiful order, checking off each item as they finish putting them down on paper. Writing for me is an act of trust, trust in some circuitry that will begin to function between my brain and my hand, so that my fingers as they click on the keyboard will make sentences that make sense. The process is linked for me to something similar in my experience of reading: I trust that I will notice something that needs to be noticed, that I am particularly suited to pick out, even though I do not know in advance what that might be.

I experienced this trust, or at least became aware of it, early in my reading and writing life. Not, to be sure, in my earliest school experiences: what I most remember from those experiences is the challenge of sounding out the words on the page and the physical effort of forming the letters, copying them over and over again in my notebook, and, at a later date, the effort of forming grammatical sentences. I doubt that I felt it at the time, but in retrospect I feel enormous gratitude to the teachers who endured what must have been the considerable tedium of imparting these lessons.

My early reading experiences were complicated somewhat by my parents' anxieties about potentially compromising my eyesight. Neither of them had had to wear eyeglasses as children, and my father, by then in his 50s, was proud of the fact that he still did not need them. There was a sense, largely unvoiced but clearly floating about in the family, that glasses were unattractive and should, if at all possible, be avoided.

DOI: 10.4324/9781003516118-3

My brother Marty, older by some five years, was praised for his perfect vision. My mother more than once recited Dorothy Parker's quip that "Men seldom make passes at girls who wear glasses." As for boys, glasses made them look like weaklings or like eggheads.

Both my parents were convinced that near-sightedness was caused by reading in poor light or simply by too much reading. My increasing absorption in books was a cause for alarm. "Turn on the light; you're going to hurt your eyes." "Enough with that book; you're going to make yourself wear glasses." "Stevie," my mother would call from the living room, "put down that book and come watch 'I Love Lucy.'" When my eyesight began to change, around the onset of puberty, I made every attempt to hide the myopia. In the backseat of our car, on a long drive to Florida, I read the road signs through binoculars in the hope that no one would notice that I couldn't make them out unaided. And when I could no longer keep up the charade, I felt shame. "Do you see what all that reading led to? We told you." Wearing my first pair of glasses on my way home from the optometrist's, I experienced acute, almost overwhelming embarrassment. I thought that everyone was looking at me, and I wanted the ground to open and swallow me up.

But writing was never associated with any of these feelings. At first it was difficult, to be sure, but there was no taint of failure, nothing shameful or embarrassing about it. On the contrary, laboriously forming the sentences and setting them down on paper was a mark of success. Later, considerably later, I began to count on the sentences coming to me. And they did. I can still recall the pleasure of writing the sentence that began one of my undergraduate papers: "All over Evelyn Waugh's England, country houses are being torn down." And still more I can conjure up the pleasure—the joy even—that came with writing the first sentence of my Ph.D. dissertation: "Sir Henry Yelverton, the king's attorney general, was no friend to Sir Walter Ralegh." I know perfectly well that there is nothing particularly remarkable about either of these sentences. Indeed there is something fatuous about confessing the auto-erotic satisfaction that came with writing them. But there it is. The satisfaction was bound up with a sense of making a modestly original opening move—at least neither sentence seemed to me entirely predictable—in the writing equivalent of a chess game. Still more, it was bound up with what I have called trust.

It strikes me as noteworthy that this trust came first in writing and only afterwards in reading. That is, it was only after I had developed some confidence in what I have called the game of writing—sitting down and allowing the sentences to form—that I developed a comparable confidence as a reader. In the 1970s, after I had already published two books (the two that in fact open with the sentences I have quoted here), I began to experience something strange and, as I felt it, thrilling. I began to read through long Renaissance works—the enormous collections of travel texts assembled by Hakluyt and Purchas, for example, or the daunting volumes of early Protestant tracts and sermons published by the Parker Society—and felt my eyes drawn to certain passages. It was as if the passages were coming to me unbidden. And I knew that I could make something of them—that is, I trusted that I could write about them.

What are the origins of such trust which might easily seem, after all, ill-founded and implausible? The likeliest analogy that comes to mind is the act of walking. It is for most of us the easiest and most ordinary ability in the world, but it is worth remembering that we were not born with it; we were taught it, and in part taught it to ourselves, through trial and error, by means of innumerable repeated experiments that we have now entirely forgotten. In taking each step there comes a moment, the moment of weight-shifting and forward-propulsion, in which we trust that we will somehow retain our balance. In the Yale Art Museum, there is a wonderful Picasso painting of a mother teaching a child to walk that perfectly captures the zany implausibility of it all.

The painting, with its mother tenderly supporting the careering toddler, also captures the crucial role played in my writing, as in my walking, by my mother. My father was a wonderfully voluble speaker, celebrated in his social circles for his flashes of merriment, his ribald jokes with their Yiddish punchlines, his ability to narrate his life as if it were a comic adventure. But in his writing he was oddly stilted and formal. My mother by contrast was shy and quiet, but whenever she encountered a serious problem, she would sit down and in her beautiful handwriting—she had been taught something called the Palmer Method—she would write it out and wrestle whatever it was into shape. I no longer recall what must have been the innumerable times that she served, like the mother in the Picasso painting, to keep me from falling on my face—but I sense her standing behind me even now when I am writing these very sentences.

Robert Pinsky

Poet

I think I remember the exact moment when I became a writer. At the age of nine I read the *Alice* books over and over. In a way, I was reading them all the time: not with the printed books in front of me, but with the stories of Alice making a small but persistent current, all day and probably in my dreams, in the stream of my attention. Reading can do that. I felt the stories purely, innocent of much distinction between a book and a movie, between a movie and a fantasy, between playing cowboys and hearing a Tom Mix cowboy episode on the radio. It was all *story*, and as a presence inside me it was all real.

My favorite passage in *Through the Looking Glass* was the story of Alice and the Fawn, in the wood where things have no names. Studying the Tenniel illustration, I was moved by the sweet awkwardness of Alice's arms clasped around the Fawn's neck as they walk together. The girl and the animal look peaceful and a little sad, as though in that paradise together they sense the moment coming soon when they will leave the wood and Alice will remember her name—she feels sure it begins with an "L."

Soon, as they leave the wood, the Fawn will cry out joyously "I'm a Fawn!" and then: "And, dear me, you're a human child!" With a "sudden look of alarm" in its "beautiful brown eyes" the Fawn runs away.

One day I decided to give myself the pleasure of reading that story again. The illustration made the page easy to find. But what I remembered like a feature-length movie was less than a page: just a few sentences I could cover with one hand! That seemed impossible, but there it was. From "Just then a Fawn came wandering by" to "it had darted away at full speed," the unforgettable episode takes only a couple of hundred words. I felt, first, a mixture of outrage and mystification. How could the book I loved trick me that way? With a few words? Then, I felt wonder. How was something so real created in such a small space? How had the writer built so much inside my

DOI: 10.4324/9781003516118-4

mind? That is a question I am still trying to answer. Reading made me need to write.

Alice feels ready to cry at having suddenly lost "her dear little fellow-traveler." Then: "'However, I know my name now,'" she said, 'that's *some* comfort.'"

In that sentence I find a great underlying truth. With Alice's understated phrase "*some* comfort," spoken to herself, Lewis Carroll invites the reader—or a certain kind of reader—into an effortful, constrained post-paradise adventure, beginning with the rudimentary but useful denotation of your name. The adventure extends into all the names for everything in the world. It may not be glorious, and it may be a kind of mourning for what has been lost, but it is, precisely, some comfort.

The passage about the wood where things have no name embodies in a specific, literal way the thrill of not being yourself. Or is it the thrill of being yourself, but in a new place or a new way, with former labels removed? Those alternatives recall the saying that there are two basic stories: someone goes on a journey; and a stranger comes to town. For readers and for writers, both stories apply as imagination explores a limitless range of departures and arrivals, exiles and immigrations.

The thrill of not being yourself includes the imagination's pleasure of being Alice and of being the Fawn and also, somehow, being the magical forest without names—the forest being yourself before words. There is also the reader's thrill of becoming the story's author. By embracing the reality of the girl and the animal on their brief, doomed journey together, the ardent reader, like a colonized country that transforms the invader, becomes a new, additional incarnation of "Lewis Carroll"—which, as Charles Dodgson's pen name, happens to be yet another creation of the writer. The story is larger than the few words that create it because the reader, absorbed and absorbing, collaborates in the action of making the setting, the characters and their action elaborately real. The reader becomes the story's co-creator—and, sometimes, becomes a writer.

"Writing" is the wrong word, speaking strictly: a misnomer for what I try to do in a poem. Maybe "composing"? The vocal work resembles noodling at a piano or squeezing clay or smooshing paint around on a surface. The physical material—the sounds, the clay, the paint, like the audible shapes of sentences, even nonsense sentences or the toddler's babble—brings you news about what you are thinking and feeling. The clay psychoanalyzes you while you play with it. At the piano, your fingers make a couple of chords that tell you about yourself. The pen or the keyboard transcribes the primary, basic reality forming in your mind's ear.

This is a theory of writing in general: it is an extension of reading. But theory aside, what about the actual practice? What in particular drives me to assemble a machine made out of words?

Possibly, I crave the stranger's excitement at entering a new village, fearful and hopeful. Or the similar feeling when you start a journey. That is, I am driven to write by loneliness, mingled with dread and attraction.

Here is a moment from Isaac Babel's "The Story of My Dovecot," in the excellent translation by Walter Morison:

> a young peasant in a waistcoat was smashing a window frame in the house of Khariton Efrusi. He was smashing it with a wooden mallet, striking out with his whole body. Sighing, he smiled all around with the amiable grin of drunkenness, sweat and spiritual power. The whole street was filled with a splitting, a snapping, the song of flying wood.

This description of one figure at one moment in an historic pogrom generates, as with the passage from *Through the Looking Glass*, a mystified empathy: a viewpoint at a remove from the scene yet also inside it, immersed in details and redolent phrases. The peasant interrupts his joyful hammering to join "a procession bearing the Cross and moving from the Municipal Building." The crowd bears aloft the portrait of "the neatly-combed Tsar" and the "inflamed old women flew on in front." The communal "spiritual power" of the scene horrifies me, and in the nature of art I am part of the scene, a reader collaborating in its creation by Isaac Babel. As with Lewis Carroll's passage of the wood where things have no names, the writer enlists the reader in realizing a truth, the "spiritual power" of the destructive, "inflamed" mob.

I've heard people say that something was so well done it made them forsake their own efforts. The opposite is true, I think. To witness a great athletic feat or to hear a great musical performance inspires emulation. It is witnessing something clumsy or false that makes one feel "why bother?". Great writing makes me want to write.

The poet William Carlos Williams looked out of his window at some roofers at work:

FINE WORK WITH PITCH AND COPPER

Now they are resting
in the fleckless light
separately in unison

like the sacks
of sifted stone stacked
regularly by twos

about the flat roof
ready after lunch
to be opened and strewn

The copper in eight
foot strips has been
beaten lengthwise

down the center at right
angles and lies ready
to edge the coping

One still chewing
picks up a copper strip
and runs his eye along it.

The poem does its work in seventy-six words, title included: about a third as long as the *Alice* episode of the wood where things have no names. Like and unlike Charles Dodgson creating Lewis Carroll creating Alice's sense that her name begins with an "L," like and unlike Isaac Babel inhabiting the terrible exaltation of the peasant celebrating the violence of a pogrom, Williams, in his poem's final three lines, catches by empathy the moment of luxurious, controlled blur between work and lunch, the roofer's casual autonomy in that borderland, inspecting the material while "still chewing."

Williams is good at noticing vernacular gestures on the fly. In "The Young Housewife," he notices how a driver can "bow and pass smiling" from the wheel. In "To a Poor Old Woman," he demonstrates that with the right kind of attention, you can see—see, with your eyes!—how plums taste to another person.

The sounds of the words help you feel that you see. Technique at that level inspires emulation. "Fine Work with Pitch and Copper" begins in the key of a short "e" sound in "resting," "fleckless" and "separately," then it modulates into the "oo" sound of "twos" and "roof" and "strewn." The middle sentence, about the copper strips, could appear in an instruction manual, or in a manual about the expert deployment of vowels and consonants and the pulsing of melody through syntax.

Williams as a teenager had *Palgrave's Golden Treasury* by heart, he has said. Like many other readers of that popular, old-fashioned anthology, he thrilled to the sounds of poems by Shakespeare, Herrick, Keats, Southey and by many now-forgotten Victorian and Edwardian poets. Reading inspires writing. At a certain pitch of intensity, reading becomes writing. Truth encourages truthfulness, attention heightens attention and art inspires art.

Jane Leavy

Biographer

Why I Write

I met Joan Didion when I was thirteen and was her dinner partner at a Manhattan restaurant that served a lot of herring. I say thirteen, but probably I was older, and only felt thirteen in her presence. In any event, I was old enough to know who she was, and what she meant to my father, Morton L. Leavy, an entertainment lawyer, who represented both Joan and her novelist husband John Gregory Dunne.

This dinner came a bit before she wrote her 1969 dispatch from Hawaii, "In the Islands," which appeared later in *The White Album*: "We are here on this island in the middle of the Pacific in lieu of filing for divorce."

That possibility, John confided later, was mitigated by their inability to decide who would get Mort in a divorce.

My father counted a whole lot of literary heavyweights among his clients: Wole Soyinka, Don DeLillo, John Irving, and John Le Carre, who slept in our den between wives and beat me six-love in tennis without relinquishing a point. I was ten.

But nothing made him prouder than handling the affairs of *Didionand-Dunne*—he favored the word handling for the intimacy it implied. Handling included managing the adoption of their daughter Quintana Roo, the sale of their Malibu house when they relocated to New York, as well as negotiating all their book and movie deals, one of which was celebrated in the August 1983 encomium John wrote for *Esquire,* in which he turned my father's name into a mantra. "Morton Leavy is short, round and benign," he wrote, like "a Jewish Dr. Doolittle"—"crossed with a pit bull," he added, not for publication.

So, I'm quite sure he didn't intend for Joan to be seated across from me at the far end of a long rectangular table in a spare Scandinavian restaurant, away from all the grownups.

What I remember most about the dinner is how sorry I felt for her at being stuck with me, that she never took off her trench coat—she was so

DOI: 10.4324/9781003516118-5

very thin, almost translucent—and her silence. She was as quiet as the negative space in her prose. Which, of course, I attributed to being stuck across the table from me. And I remember a smorgasbord as spare as a Didion sentence.

She had not yet written "Why I Write" for the *New York Times*, a title she stole from George Orwell, in which she said: "I write entirely to find out what I'm thinking."

I had not yet realized I, too, was a writer.

I had not yet escaped academia and a misbegotten collegiate foray into Renaissance iconography and the music of the spheres. I had not figured out that I could get paid to write by the word, which when you get right down to it is a compelling reason to do anything. I had not yet been hired by the *Washington Post* to write sports and features. I had not signed a contract to write my first novel, blurbed by John Gregory Dunne. I had not yet suffered my first case of writer's block, a neurological spasm dismissed by my father with a terse tautological imperative: "Writers write." I was gratified to learn he told Joan the same thing.

I had not yet endured the infuriating suggestion *why don't you make an outline?* Each time, I thanked Joan before replying, *how can I make an outline when I don't know what I think?*

Some seventeen years after that dinner, after finding a place and a voice at the *Washington Post*, my first child arrived, and I took a year-long leave from the paper. For the first time in my adult life, I had nothing to write, no beat to cover, no deadlines to meet, except those involving diapers.

It was disorienting not to know what I thought. Worse, I began to question who I was.

I signed on as an adjunct professor at Georgetown University to teach journalism to juniors and seniors. But they didn't know how to spell Puerto Rico or Marion Barry, so the curriculum quickly evolved into a class in remedial writing. I made them read Didion and diagram her sentences, the grammar that imposed structure on thought. I made them read "Why I Write," emphasizing the part where Didion says,

> In many ways writing is the act of saying *I*, of imposing oneself upon other people, of saying *listen to me, see it my way, change your mind*. It's an aggressive, even a hostile act . . . the tactic of a secret bully.

She carefully eschewed the psychoanalytic term, but helped me to understand that the diminution of ego I felt in the absence of writing meant losing my sense of myself.

Ordinarily, I do not think about Sigmund Freud when I sit down to write. The only exception was when I tried to shoehorn his complaint about meager literary royalties into my biography of Babe Ruth. I could not find a place for the letter he wrote to his nephew in New York complaining about his publisher, but I never felt more well-disposed to him, either.

I know that the mastery of physical feats—hitting a baseball or driving a car, for example—begins as a cognitive act: first you do this, then you do that. That after you incorporate something into your mental apparatus and do it routinely, it becomes implicit rather than explicit. I know that when athletes are called upon to reverse that process, to explain themselves and what they do in words, mastery is compromised. They falter. They swing and miss. A serve goes long.

I think about this a lot when I am stuck in my writing. When I can't find exactly the right word. Sometimes I have to revert to pen and paper, often in the middle of the night when the sentence finally comes, wafting into consciousness on a gust of REM sleep. Sometimes I have to take a shower. The water seems to help.

Despite what you may think, this summoning is a visceral process. Nauseating even.

Later, when there's time, if the ink hasn't bled into whatever scrap of paper I've seized to get the words down before they evaporate, I may wonder about the neurological alchemy that leads from brain to fingers on a keyboard.

That moment of actualization is incendiary. As when my grandmother leaned into the oven to hold a wooden match to the pilot light to bake my rugelach, and the cold jets set in cast iron caught with a whoosh of warmth, a whiff of Sulphur, a flash of illumination that settled almost as quickly as it had ignited. It is thrilling, addictive even.

Why do writers write? It's like asking why alcoholics drink.

I last saw Joan at a November 11, 2011, book event in Washington for *Blue Nights*, her grieving sequel about Quintana Roo's descent into fatal illness. The first volume, a bestseller and a play starring Vanessa Redgrave, *The Year of Magical Thinking*, had described John's death upon returning home from visiting Quintana in the first of four Intensive Care Units in which she spent too much of the last twenty months of her life.

In lieu of a reading, the publisher had organized a Q & A with Susan Stamberg of National Public Radio at a formerly grand movie house with a painted mural in the ceiling's dome showing the god Mercury casting a reel of film across the sky to a cherub. The publisher also commissioned a fifteen-minute promotional film for which Joan had recorded the first two chapters of the book. It was a brilliant strategy because nobody, not even Joan Didion, could have read that aloud to strangers again and again.

I noticed she never took off her trench coat.

In the film, directed by her nephew Griffin Dunne, the Manhattan skyline appears dirge blue, like Joan's voice, narrating her journey through crowded East Side intersections into Central Park and out of it again, the sky and her voice lightening only upon arriving at St. John the Divine, the great cathedral in upper Manhattan, for Quintana's wedding. There's the bride exiting a limousine on sunny Amsterdam Avenue, engulfed by young attendants draped in the Hawaiian leis she had requested. The bride and groom kneeling in cool darkness by the altar. The nuclear family gathering in the cathedral house for the cutting of the cake.

"Peach-colored from Payard," Joan read.

A black and white photograph commemorates the moment: the bride in white and in profile, her parents in large sunglasses commanding the center, and at the far right, at the edge of the frame, at the edge of consciousness, my father photo-bombing the wedding party.

The image came and went before I could be certain. What was he doing there? Mostly deaf and largely blind, he was no longer handling their affairs.

"The date was July 26, 2003," Joan read.

That was the last time he left the house. He was dead five weeks later.

To see him on the big screen above Joan's shoulder, eight years later, alive in the millisecond between coming and going, was thrilling and crushing—like finding the right word and losing it.

Recently, during a particularly fallow time in my writing life, two years without making sentences, I found on Netflix the full-length documentary Griffin Dunne made about his aunt Joan. It's called "The Center Will Not Hold," a line she used to describe Haight-Ashbury in the Sixties. A line that describes me without writing.

I paused the film at the tableau of the wedding cake: yes, it was my father. I ran it back and forth to make sure and took a screenshot, too. Each time he appeared brought the adrenaline rush I feel every time I find the right word and hang onto it.

Each time, I hear him say, "Writers write." And I know who I am.

Joseph Leo Koerner

Art Historian and Filmmaker

Woodland Road

Some years ago, before my mother died, I returned to Pittsburgh to open an exhibition of my father's paintings at Chatham University. The tiny show—ten pictures in a student common room repurposed as gallery space—had been thrust on Chatham by Beth, a high school friend. Beth had admired my father's paintings ever since she saw them densely hung on the walls of my childhood home. To minimize costs, all but one of the exhibited paintings came from that home, where my mother still lived, piously curating my father's extensive artistic remains.

The exhibition's only proper loan was from a neighborhood bank. When it was a flourishing civic institution, the Squirrel Hill branch of Pittsburgh National Bank purchased *Man on the Pole* for its front office. Since the seventies, my father's painting has hung on the wall behind the row of teller counters, beside the gleaming steel door to the bank's vault. Like the other works in the show, that canvas was of Pittsburgh and painted in Pittsburgh. It depicted an outsize repairman on a telephone pole above Bigelow Boulevard, with a vista of the Strip District behind and a TV camera operator on a Chapman crane filming the action. We borrowed *Man on Pole* because Beth thought it would be wise to include at least one work that Pittsburghers could have possibly seen in a public setting.

The other pictures were chosen for their connection to Chatham. All were painted during my father's artist-in-residency in 1952–53, when Chatham University was still the Pennsylvania College for Women. My mother was a sophomore there, studying to be an orchestra musician. Spotting her in a practice room, and liking her bobbed blonde hair, my father portrayed her placing her violin into its case. A year later, my parents married, and when my sister arrived in 1954, my mother put the violin away for good. Part of family history, Chatham also changed the direction of my father's art. After twelve years of painting from drawings and photographs in his studio, first in war-torn Berlin, then in Brooklyn,

DOI: 10.4324/9781003516118-6

he began—at Chatham, with scores of undergrads eager to pose for him—to work always and only from life, and in a manner modeled on paintings by Paul Cézanne.

On the evening before the show's opening Beth organized a dinner at the home of a wealthy donor. The big Arts and Crafts-style residence was familiar to me. On the highest stretch of Woodland Road—the leafy drive, just blocks from my home, that winds its way through Chatham's undulating campus—the house had been part of my morning paper route. Entering the dark oak door at which, decades earlier, I aimed rolled-up copies of the *Pittsburgh Post-Gazette*, I was greeted by a festive display. On a decorative bentwood easel erected in the middle of the entrance hall stood a framed canvas painting about three feet wide. Approaching the display, with guests drawing close in expectant silence, I recognized it as a work by my father's hand. Indeed, the picture was a most intimate acquaintance. It had been painted with me, my sister, and my mother all present throughout the three long days of its execution out-of-doors, in the southern reaches of the Vienna Woods.

"That's the pig lady in Lainzer Tiergarten!" I exclaimed, laughing. "Where in the world did you get it?"

Taking his place beside the easel, the host replied: "It's not mine. It's my brother's. He lent it just for tonight. He hoped you might answer a question. He wanted to know what it means."

"What what means?"

"The painting. People always ask him what it means, and he has no idea. So, he wanted me to ask you, to find out if you know."

"Well, I'm not sure what it means, but I can tell you exactly what it is," I began cheerfully. "It's a painting of an old lady way less than five feet tall who used to feed bread rolls to the wild boars. The boars rampaged in great droves through that big walled-in section of the Wienerwald—the Vienna Woods. The young ones were incredibly cute, with striping for camouflage, as you can see," said I, pointing to the several piglets in the foreground, their white, brown, and tan fur carefully rendered by the flat edge of my father's square-tipped brush. "The two big brown ones on the right are sows, adult females. They can be super vicious when hungry or cornered, or when they're protecting their young. You can see the woman, the pig lady, has a big stick to beat the pigs if they get too aggressive. We thought it was so bizarre, this tiny woman stirring up these animals into a feeding frenzy, then clubbing them on the nose if they fought over the bread. She hit them if they acted piggy, but it was her bread rolls that riled them up! My mother, who was herself rather small, was terrified even by littlest piglets, especially when it rained, because rain made them restless. If you ran, they ran towards you and with you, dozens of them, with their mothers crashing through the bushes to join in the race. But the pig lady—that's what my sister and I called her—she was fearless and cruel, a merciless disciplinarian of the pigs. And she fed them literally every day, rain or shine, with day-old bread from a local bakery, and always carrying her walking stick."

My host, observing me closely, seemed unsatisfied, so I went on.

"You see, this is the sort of thing my father chose to paint. Something strange that he didn't invent, but that he—actually, our whole family—chanced upon while walking. And walking was what we mostly did in Vienna every summer, all summer long. The Lainzer Tiergarten is a fenced wildlife preserve completely overrun by wild boar, although it is supposed to contain some rare animals, like mouflon and elks. Originally it served as hunting grounds for the ruling Habsburg family—the dream castle of Empress Elisabeth, of 'Sissy,' is a museum on the grounds. We never saw mouflon or elk. Only boar. But we loved them, especially the young piglets, and also the huge, tusked solitary males that lurked in the deep forest. Rarely seen, they could be heard from far away rooting in the soil. Maybe we liked the boar because my mother was so afraid of them and that they made us feel brave. And we liked to spot the pig lady, too, as if she were an elusive specimen, like the mighty horned mouflon hidden in the woods. We made up stories about the woman's homelife and mimicked the curses she muttered as she wacked the boars for being greedy. We squirmed with embarrassment when he approached her, but we were happy when my father convinced the pig lady to pose for your painting."

Feeling my audience was growing restless, I endeavored to conclude.

"I guess I should say we children were always involved in his paintings. Not just when he painted us, which was often, especially when we did something interesting-looking, like climbing a wall and pretending to be a statue or placing odd things on our head and parading before him. In Vienna we were a grumpy team of four, with my father the leader and only German-speaker, and my mother, way younger than he, and cautious and practical, calculating lunch stops and how to get home from remote places, like the gate at the southernmost corner of the Tiergarten, where no trains or busses stopped, and we hitchhiked back to town. June through September we wandered Vienna, my father's childhood home, while he painted or drew along the way, creating works he'd sell back in Pittsburgh. That's how he made his living. Painting pictures like this one of the pig lady and selling them to people like your brother, I guess."

This was not what our host wanted to hear, and the more detailed my story became, the stranger the painting began to seem. Resembling in style, colors, and format an ordinary Impressionist landscape, and framed for formal display in an elegant living room, it suddenly became a mortifying intruder, the one thing in this household that clearly did not belong.

Changing tack, I began again.

"My father's undertaking was odd, and it seemed odd even to me as a child. Only he, it seemed, marched through the Wienerwald regularly, year after year, searching for things to paint, and with a whole family in tow. And even if there had been a Sunday painter out for a walk in the woods, he or she would never have planted themselves before the pig lady, never posed her for hours at a time feeding and repelling the pigs. Something inexplicable drove him to paint what he did in the way he did. And the way he painted was to let his subjects—his 'motifs,' as he called them—come unplanned to him. Asked what one of his picture's meant, he'd usually answer (excuse the language): 'What the fuck do you think it means?' The pig lady was my obsession more than my father's. But when I think about why I found her so compelling, I imagine it was because I thought my father would paint her, and I wanted to be in on the action. From all those walks, and all the drawings and paintings he made on them, I knew what he liked to paint. But I didn't know why he painted what he did, so I can't explain what his pictures mean.

In retrospect, if I were forced to say, I would wager that she, the pig lady in Lainzer Tiergarten, represented all the Viennese of her generation bundled together, all the embittered war widows who populated the desolate, formerly Jewish neighborhood where my father was born, and where he insisted we live: poor lonely pensioners we never got to know personally, traveling, as we did, incognito, as our self-enclosed, English-speaking unit of four. She was, for example, the ill-tempered Hausbesorgerin Frau Lange, the cleaning lady slash building manager who patrolled the apartment block we lived in. Smelling richly of urine, she screamed at everyone for tiny infractions committed, say, when emptying trash. She was the short, stout greengrocer who, for years the friendliest of vendors, suddenly out of nowhere refused our patronage, muttering curses and spitting at us as we left her shop. She was the Viennese neighbor who, in 1938, when Hitler arrived, kicked Jews like my father's family out of the apartments they'd been living in for generations, to be sent by train to the east, to places near Riga and Minsk, to be shot or gassed upon arrival. She was all that pent-up enmity and rage shrunk down to the size of us children, and turned into something comical, inscrutable, and dangerous all at once. That's why the painting looks strange where it stands. It's about home, about my father's Viennese home, as an uncanny place. It's about what Sigmund Freud, a Viennese like my father, who escaped from his home in 1938—it's what Freud called 'das Unheimliche.' That word doesn't translate well into English, because the German means both the homely and the unhomely, both the deeply familiar and the terrifying and uncanny. The painting wants to belong, but it can't, not here in this house, not tomorrow in the gallery in Chatham, not in any history of art. It's too conventional and too strange, I guess."

I wish I could report that *this* is what drives me to write. That I write to escape such awkward moments as the one which occurred on Woodland Road, and as happened to me earlier and often while growing up, when friends visiting my home would ask me to explain the strange paintings on the walls. I wish I could say that such experiences drove me to write about well-known artists of the past in a conviction that they, the old masters, were right about suffering—"no document of civilization is not at the same time a document of barbarism," et cetera. Whatever drives it, however, writing never reached the pig lady—how she entered the walled Tiergarten through her own private iron gate, how she behaved towards my father with malicious deference, knowing exactly what sort of Viennese revenant he was. How she never once so much as glanced at me. How she bludgeoned me, her dedicated scribe, with perfect indifference.

Josh Ritter

Singer, Songwriter, Musician, Novelist

TRUTH IS A DIMENSION (BOTH INVISIBLE AND BLINDING)

I GOT OFF THE HIGHWAY NORTH OF DESERT CANYON STATION
WAS DRIVIN WITH MY HEADLIGHTS OFF JUST STARS FOR
NAVIGATION
MY TELESCOPE MY NOTES MY HAM SANDWICHES AND COFFEE
SOMETIMES YOU MUST BE ALL ALONE THERE AIN'T NO WAY TO
NOT BE

I WAS THINKING ABOUT TONYA HOW THINGS HAD
REARRANGED
AND EVERYTHING HAD GONE FULL CIRCLE WE WERE BACK TO
BEING STRANGERS
SHE WAS WITH A MAN NAMED NEIL NOW THAT'S ALL I KNEW
ABOUT HIM
I WAS HAPPY SHE WAS HAPPY REAL HAPPY THAT SHE'D
FOUND HIM

IT WAS JUST AFTER ELEVEN WHEN I PULLED OFF AT THE
LOOKOUT
THE PARKING LOT WAS EMPTY THOUGH THE AIR STILL
SMELLED LIKE COOKOUTS
AND YES I ADMIT I TOKED ONE BUT THAT DOESN'T CHANGE
WHAT HAPPENED
AND ANYWAY YOU'RE NOT MY PARENTS AND IT REALLY HELPS
MY MAPPING

OF THE SYSTEM 611 A MAGELLANIC CLUSTER
I'D BEEN WATCHING FOR AWHILE I GOT MY TELESCOPE
ADJUSTED

DOI: 10.4324/9781003516118-7

AND I TURNED IT TOWARD AN UNASSUMING PATCH OF
   DUSTY SKY
THAT WAS REALLY FIFTY MILLION STARS A BILLION LIGHT
   YEARS WIDE

THEN ALL AT ONCE IT FELT AS IF TIME HAD BEEN SUSPENDED
AND A VISION POURED INTO ME LIKE A BOTTLE'D BEEN
   UPENDED
I WAS FILLED WITH REVELATION BOTH INFINITE AND FINITE
THAT FILTERED DOWN MY TELESCOPE ENCODED IN THE
   STARLIGHT

IT SAID, '*TRUTH IS NOT IMMUTABLE BUT ITSELF IS
   A DIMENSION
TRUTH CAN BE BOTH WEIGHTED DOWN AND WARPED IN
   STRANGE DIRECTIONS
TRUTH HAS A SHAPE THAT ALTERS EACH ACCORDING TO
   OBSERVER
SOMETIMES YOU MUST BE CLOSE TO IT SOMETIMES YOU MUST
   BE FURTHER*

*TRUTH CAN BEND AND TRUTH CAN BREAK DEPENDS ON
   HOW YOU ASK IT
IT FRAYS OR IT MAY BLAZE OUT AT SOME PAUL BOUND FOR
   DAMASCUS
IT SOMETIMES GETS MISTOOK FOR GOD SOMETIMES FOR ITS
   SERVANT
IT BOTH EXISTS AND DOESN'T LIKE A STAR THAT'S NOT
   OBSERVED YET'*

WHICH ALL AT ONCE RETURNED MY THOUGHTS TO
   SYSTEM 611
STILL TWINKLING DOWN THE TELESCOPE INTO MY MIND
   FROM HEAVEN
AND I STOOD THERE LOOKING UPWARD AS THE DARKNESS
   TURNED TO DAWN
AND RECEIVED THAT STRANGE TRANSMISSION UNTIL FINALLY
   IT WAS GONE

AND I KNEW BEYOND A SHADOW MY DISCOVERY WAS REAL
BUT THE PERSON THAT I LONGED TO TELL WAS SOUND ASLEEP
   WITH NEIL
IN SOME PARALLEL DIMENSION MAYBE TONYA WAS STILL MINE

BUT IN THIS ONE SHE STILL LOVED HIM AND THAT LEFT ME TO
    SEARCH THE SKY

SO I WROTE THIS PAPER TO ALERT YOU TO MY FINDINGS
I CALL IT 'TRUTH IS A DIMENSION BOTH INVISIBLE AND
    BLINDING'
YOU CAN GIVE ME THE AWARDS NOW YOU CAN KNIGHT ME
    OR WHATEVER
I'VE GOT NOTHING GOING ON NOW ME AND TONYA AREN'T
    TOGETHER

GO AHEAD AND LAUGH AT ME AND ALL OF MY
    CONCLUSIONS
IN SYMPOSIUMS AND SEMINARS AND THINK TANK
    INSTITUTIONS
YOU MAY EVEN TALK TO TONYA LET ME ASK YOU IF YOU DO
PLEASE TELL HER I STILL LOVE HER THAT WILL ALWAYS
    BE THE TRUTH.

Nicole Sealey

Poet

Expect to be Sung to: Brigit Pegeen Kelly's "Song"

Listen . . .

Samuel Taylor Coleridge once described poetry as "the best words in the best order." While Coleridge's claim may betray a certain bias and come across as overly generous, what I think he meant is that the best *poetry* is comprised of the best words in the best order.

Poems are part-skill, part-magic and all mystery. Though we can't speak to the magic and mystery with any real authority, apart from the importance of being present to receive said magic and being open to said mysteries, we can speak to the matter of craft. The skill part. What better way for students of poetry, of which I will always be, to learn craft than to examine the poems that we hold dear? To explore poems that drive us to write?

"Song" by Brigit Pegeen Kelly is one such poem, universally admired for its greatness. If you're not familiar with the poem, I won't hold that against you but rather envy you, as you're in for a treat. Here's "Song":

Listen: there was a goat's head hanging by ropes in a tree.
All night it hung there and sang. And those who heard it
Felt a hurt in their hearts and thought they were hearing
The song of a night bird. They sat up in their beds, and then
They lay back down again. In the night wind, the goat's head
Swayed back and forth, and from far off it shone faintly
The way the moonlight shone on the train track miles away
Beside which the goat's headless body lay. Some boys
Had hacked its head off. It was harder work than they had imagined.
The goat cried like a man and struggled hard. But they
Finished the job. They hung the bleeding head by the school
And then ran off into the darkness that seems to hide everything.
The head hung in the tree. The body lay by the tracks.
The head called to the body. The body to the head.

DOI: 10.4324/9781003516118-8

They missed each other. The missing grew large between them,
Until it pulled the heart right out of the body, until
The drawn heart flew toward the head, flew as a bird flies
Back to its cage and the familiar perch from which it trills.
Then the heart sang in the head, softly at first and then louder,
Sang long and low until the morning light came up over
The school and over the tree, and then the singing stopped . . .
The goat had belonged to a small girl. She named
The goat Broken Thorn Sweet Blackberry, named it after
The night's bush of stars, because the goat's silky hair
Was dark as well water, because it had eyes like wild fruit.
The girl lived near a high railroad track. At night
She heard the trains passing, the sweet sound of the train's horn
Pouring softly over her bed, and each morning she woke
To give the bleating goat his pail of warm milk. She sang
Him songs about girls with ropes and cooks in boats.
She brushed him with a stiff brush. She dreamed daily
That he grew bigger, and he did. She thought her dreaming
Made it so. But one night the girl didn't hear the train's horn,
And the next morning she woke to an empty yard. The goat
Was gone. Everything looked strange. It was as if a storm
Had passed through while she slept, wind and stones, rain
Stripping the branches of fruit. She knew that someone
Had stolen the goat and that he had come to harm. She called
To him. All morning and into the afternoon, she called
And called. She walked and walked. In her chest a bad feeling
Like the feeling of the stones gouging the soft undersides
Of her bare feet. Then somebody found the goat's body
By the high tracks, the flies already filling their soft bottles
At the goat's torn neck. Then somebody found the head
Hanging in a tree by the school. They hurried to take
These things away so that the girl would not see them.
They hurried to raise money to buy the girl another goat.
They hurried to find the boys who had done this, to hear
Them say it was a joke, a joke, it was nothing but a joke . . .
But listen: here is the point. The boys thought to have
Their fun and be done with it. It was harder work than they
Had imagined, this silly sacrifice, but they finished the job,
Whistling as they washed their large hands in the dark.
What they didn't know was that the goat's head was already
Singing behind them in the tree. What they didn't know
Was that the goat's head would go on singing, just for them,
Long after the ropes were down, and that they would learn to listen,
Pail after pail, stroke after patient stroke. They would

Wake in the night thinking they heard the wind in the trees
Or a night bird, but their hearts beating harder. There
Would be a whistle, a hum, a high murmur, and, at last, a song,
The low song a lost boy sings remembering his mother's call.
Not a cruel song, no, no, not cruel at all. This song
Is sweet. It is sweet. The heart dies of this sweetness.

This poem gets me every time, and I selfishly manufacture occasions to read, talk or write about it—case in point.

The first word of the poem, "listen," is a direct command. Unlike the verb "hear," inherent in "listen" is to *hear for understanding*. The poem asks not just for our ears but also for our attention. The command is followed by the image of "a goat's head hanging by ropes in a tree." A hard stop ends the line, giving readers time to register the horror. The second sentence recalls, without spectacle, the dismembered goat's head singing. The night wind blowing the goat's head back and forth calls up the image and sound of a wind chime, albeit a nightmarish one.

Titles create expectations that poems can meet, fall short of or, in some cases, intentionally undermine. With Kelly's "Song," readers expect to be sung to. The poem not only makes mention to song, singing, whistling, etcetera, it also makes good use of rhyme, rhythm, anaphora, alliteration, etcetera—all the elements of a *good* song. Take, for instance, the slant rhymes "hurt," "hearts" and "thoughts" in the lines: "And those who heard it/Felt a hurt in their hearts and thought they were hearing/ The song of a night bird." Further, because Kelly balances traditionally clichéd language with strange imagery, the phrase "hurt in their hearts" reads like new. The skill part.

Through an omniscient speaker, Kelly takes us from the tree, from which the goat head hangs, to the train tracks in a single beat, via moonlight:

In the night wind, the goat's head
Swayed back and forth, and from far off it shone faintly
The way the moonlight shone on the train track miles away
Beside which the goat's headless body lay.

Note the rhyme: "way," "away" and "lay." Following that complex sentence with single-syllable rhymes are simple ones: "Some boys/Had hacked its head off. It was harder work than they had imagined." The hard *h* and *a* sounds are unrelenting, like, I imagine, the sound of actual hacking. The skill part. Strategically placed complex and simple sentences slow down or speed up the poem's pace and simplify or further complicate the narrative.

The boys hung the goat's head by the school for all to see and then ran into "the darkness that seems to hide everything." The darkness is described not for what it *is* but for what it can do. Kelly uses what readers already know about the dark to infer what happens therein. The skill part. Five simple sentences follow: "The head hung in the tree. The body lay by the tracks./The head called to the body. The body to the head./They missed each other." Alternating between "head" and "body," and then including both words in subsequent sentences, emphasizes dismemberment and communicates longing, respectively. Then, magic happens:

The missing grew large between them,
Until it pulled the heart right out of the body, until
The drawn heart flew toward the head, flew as a bird flies.

There's nothing excessive about "the heart flew as a bird flies." It is perfectly plain and works precisely because of its plainness. Again, shopworn phrases are elevated by the strangeness that surrounds them. The skill part.

The ellipsis that comes after "then the singing stopped" transports us to a time before the goat's disappearance: "The goat had belonged to a small girl. She named/the goat Broken Thorn Sweet Blackberry . . ." This digression gives us insight into the goat's life. "Broken Thorn Sweet Blackberry" alludes to the fate that would befall the goat and speaks to the age of the small girl—one assumes that only a child would name a pet so whimsically. The nursery rhyme-like quality further suggests her age (i.e. "She sang/Him songs about girls with ropes and cooks in boats"). Again, because the recurring image of the goat's head is startling, other images can be less so. The goat's hair can be "dark as well water." Its eyes "like wild fruit."

"Song" continues:

At night
She heard the train passing, the sweet sound of the train's horn
Pouring softly over her bed and each morning she woke
To give the bleating goat his pail of warm milk.

The "bleating goat" is reminiscent of the "bleeding head" in the earlier line: "They hung the bleeding head by the school." "Pouring" is an odd way to describe the spread of sound, which might be why the word is situated in the same sentence as the act of the small girl giving her goat milk. The choice of "pouring" becomes less curious and more appropriate when applied to both the train's horn and the feeding. The skill part. Later lines do similar work: "Then somebody found the goat's body/By the high tracks, the flies already filling their soft bottles/At the goat's torn neck." A play on bottle flies, the word "bottles" echoes the word "body," which precedes it.

As quickly as such moments of intimacy between the girl and the goat appear, they are gone: "But one night the girl didn't hear the train's horn,/And the next morning she woke to an empty yard. The goat/Was gone. Everything looked strange." Instead of relying on "strange" to modify the morning, strangeness is qualified with the following: "It was as if a storm/Had passed through while she slept, wind and stones, rain/Stripping the branches of fruit" and "In her chest a bad feeling/Like the feeling of the stones gouging the soft undersides/Of her bare feet." "The" before "stones" gives "stones" a specificity it would lack otherwise and places "gouging" in the immediate present. Readers feel as though we're walking alongside the girl. Readers are reminded of the poem's opening a third of the way through with "But listen: here is the point." This time, however, the imperative is preceded by a conjunction, signaling a divergence from the poem's previous song, signaling the final turn. The skill part.

Upon Brigit Pegeen Kelly's death, Amie Whittemore, a former student of hers, wrote:

> I wish I could give you more of Brigit. I wish you could bask in her presence, I wish you could listen to her read a poem, enjoy her dark and roving humor, her bright mind, her warmth—though she was not affectionate. I once tried to hug her and it felt like a violation; she was as private as a diary. I think of a bird's wing, covering its body in sleep. You want to know the hard, clear soul of Brigit Pegeen Kelly? Read her poems.

This, I believe, is sound advice. But listen, here is the point: *If*, rather, *when* you decide to read more of Kelly, begin with a reread of "Song," an inspiration among poets because of its magic and mysteries. Because of its skill. It is "not a cruel song, no, no, not cruel at all. This song/Is sweet. It is sweet. The heart dies of this sweetness."

Permissions Line: Brigit Pegeen Kelly, excerpt from "Song" from *Song: Poems*. Copyright © 1995 by Brigit Pegeen Kelly. Reprinted with the permission of The Permissions Company, LLC on behalf of BOA Editions Ltd., boaeditions.org.

Patricia Churchland

Neurophilosopher

Buffaloed

My dad left the farm when he was twelve to begin working as a "print-er's devil" for a small-town newspaper, *The Brooks Bulletin,* in Alberta. Further schooling was not available. As a toddler, he suffered a bout of polio that weakened one leg so that he had a limp and could not run. Consequently, he was not suited for the otherwise likely jobs of wrangling cattle or logging or joining the army. In a favored cliché, he would say that "printer's ink was in his veins." Indeed he did know the printing trade well, from how to fix the temperamental linotype machine that melted the lead and dimpled out the lead type to how to write engagingly about erecting a telephone line over the Monashee mountains. I saw his expertise because he opened a village newspaper in British Columbia's Okanagan Valley. After school I would often stop by the *Oliver News* office to sniff the heady smell of printer's ink, or eavesdrop as the local Mountie listed the lock-ups after brawls in the beer parlor.

As children do, I began to imitate my father. I thought writing was fun. While some school tasks seemed a bit tedious, it was generally fun to write, especially if I could go beyond the bare facts and stray into some pretend facts. Once I reached high school age, I was permitted to use my dad's home typewriter, a 1928 Underwood. It was a hallowed thing. As I now use a computer, his Underwood sits on a hall table, a reminder of nights of key-pounding while the northern lights flickered outside.

I studied philosophy in college, under the misapprehension that cur-rent philosophers were trying to understand how the mind works. It took me a while to fathom that they were actually interested only in words, not things. They staged little contests where flamboyant clever-ness in wordplay counted as progress. Eventually, I made a shift away from the sterility of contemporary philosophy in favor of the vibrancy of neuroscience. I thought of myself as a "neurophilosopher," and began

DOI: 10.4324/9781003516118-9

writing about what neuroscience teaches us concerning "big-question" philosophy—questions about knowledge and morality. Feeding my passion to understand, I greedily consumed discoveries about how brains learn and love and joke. However hard-nosed my analysis of what I learned, this inference seemed increasingly plain: I am as I am because my *brain*—with its genes and neurons and experiences—is as *it* is. Recalling my father's tranquil way with logic and clarity, I suppose my writing voice, such as it is, was largely acquired around the kitchen stove and in the cow barn, as well as in *The Oliver News*.

Reporting local news, though enjoyable, is not my brief. My dad's editorial slant, however, figures in my focus inasmuch as I tend to veer toward large themes that matter to a scientifically curious community, *very* broadly construed. Why, for example, can tall tales be more appealing to people than the practical truth they urgently need? Why are we so eager to be scammed? As I child, I watched with alarm as one neighbor chose faith healing when surgery would have worked. I remain buffaloed by the fondness for voodoo over science. Moreover, as an academic, I discovered that such partiality for magic is by no means restricted to those bereft of fancy college degrees.

A recent fashion among some philosophers is to venerate a hunch that consciousness is a fundamental feature of the universe, along with charge, mass and spin—properties of electrons. I am not making this up. For these philosophers, consciousness is not the outcome of any process in our brains. Consequently, they claim that nothing about consciousness can be learned by studying the brain. This opinion is speculation, and philosophers of the "no-brain" persuasion flaunt their lack of evidence; they revere instead their intuition that conscious experience looks so utterly and fundamentally different from the physical nature of the brain that it cannot possibly emerge from such a substrate. Why seek evidence for the obvious?

This story line has a familiar resonance. Where have we heard it before? Well, regarding ideas about the nature of *life*—of livingness. According to vitalism, livingness itself cannot possibly emerge from *dead* molecules. Life requires vital spirit. Obviously. Dead is dead and living is living. The living have vital spirit, the dead do not.

As a student in a rural high school, I was lucky enough to have a sincere vitalist teach us biology (arrogant snot-heads that we students were, we lampooned his vitalism at every chance). In fact, vitalists were not uncommon, until 1953. In that year, James Watson and Francis Crick figured out the helical structure of DNA, using data from Rosalind Franklin. They showed how the very structure of the DNA molecule embodied a code using four bases; DNA codes for the proteins that make up living organisms, including us. DNA was soon recognized to be the key to heredity, and, with its chance modifications, the key to evolutionary change.

Although a few vitalists clung to their vital spirit, cell biologists continued to make progress with new microscopes and new techniques. They figured out how proteins are assembled in cells by structures called ribosomes, which take DNA code as input. They discovered how cellular structures—mitochondria—produce energy to keep living cells living. Collectively, these and related discoveries in microbiology left not a crumb for vital spirit. Replaced by molecular biology, vitalism is now regarded as an historical curiosity.

The aroma of vitalism permeates panpsychism. According to panpsychism, *everything* in the universe, including subatomic particles and cow pies, is conscious. A foretaste of this contemporary conviction can be found in the work of the Greek philosopher Thales (624–545 BC). Bewildered by just about all processes—storms, seasons, dreaming, healing—Thales threw up his hands and conceded: "everything is full of gods." Not a bad hunch, for ancient times.

So, what motivates today's panpsychists? They are bewildered by conscious phenomena, and oddly, their bewilderment gives rise to an unshakeable certainty: "can you imagine a mechanism whereby the brain might produce consciousness? No—you cannot. No one can." Taking their failure of imagination as an unequaled scientific clue, panpsychists deny the very possibility that physical brains can produce subjective experience. Consciousness must be a fundamental feature of the universe. Everything is full of gods.

Physicists, not surprisingly, typically scoff at the idea that well-behaved physical laws characterizing elementary particles such as electrons need to be revised because electrons are *conscious*. The scoffing is not about a lack of remaining puzzles about subatomic physics. Rather, physicists realize that none of the existing puzzles have anything remotely to do with conscious experience. The puzzles are at the wrong temporal scale and the wrong spatial scale. Electrons, moreover, have no components and no structure. What is there for consciousness to fit into?

Why then do "no-brain" philosophers put so much stock in what they cannot imagine? After all, what you can imagine is a rather humdrum psychological fact about you. It depends on your level of ignorance, your level of learning, and maybe the flexibility of your personality. If you know no physics, it is easy to imagine traveling faster than the speed of light, though such a speed is now known to be a physical impossibility. If you know no neuroscience, it may be impossible to imagine how the brain remembers long-past events. But that inability to imagine is not of a piece with scientific evidence about what is probably true. It is not a productive scientific clue about anything, save one's ignorance.

Perhaps no-brain philosophers just need to practice saying, "I do not know; maybe someday we will."

While a printer's devil, my dad was given a nook in the print shop where he slept. Once he found a copy of Darwin's *Origin of Species* on a bookshelf, and with little to do in off hours, he read. And read. Creationist accounts of human origins slunk off as he came to see them as preposterous. Intentional selection by farmers for horse lines that bred true also weighed against creationism. Having mulled over *The Origin of Species*, my dad later echoed Darwin's point that selective breeding is just a fast human way of doing what an ecology does slowly and without purpose. It is why polar bears are white and beavers have ever-growing teeth.

Our regular Sunday dinners with neighbors were often followed by drawn-out disagreements about whether biological mechanisms are replacing gods, and whether that replacement is desirable. When the conversation got testy, folks hauled out their violins and gathered around the piano. We all danced.

Another frequent theme of our after-dinner debates was the range of scientific surprises, such as *invisible* germs that cause infections. Such realities eventually ease their way into common sense and lose their shock value. As scientists probe reality, their written explanations—in physics, chemistry and elsewhere—may clash with everyday intuitions. Consider your scientific introduction to temperature: "In hot water, molecules are moving faster than in cold water, and that is what water temperature *is*—'kinetic energy of the constituent molecules.'" Really? Isn't heat all about hotness itself? Nope. Hotness is molecular *movement*. Or consider Copernicus in 1543: "the Earth moves around the Sun." Oh, come on! The Roman Inquisition: "This is foolish, absurd and heretical since it contradicts the Bible." They had a point. Casual observation suggests it is the Sun that moves and the Earth is stationary. Dead obvious. The veiled joy is that the dead obvious is so often dead wrong. This is also true of the brain.

Neuroscience is, in fact, making progress in understanding the structure and function of brains, bit by bit, no-brain philosophers notwithstanding. No one can tell from here how much will ultimately be explained or what concepts will be used. The human brain might be more complicated than it is smart. Nevertheless, new tools are coming online, as are new ways of saying what brains are actually up to. We see the emergence of engineering concepts that surprise our everyday intuitions about learning and perception. Many puzzles about how brains work are really deep and really tough. Such as: how are motor and cognitive skills learned and retained and performed; how can we so swiftly recollect our first kiss; how are decisions made? The list of mysteries is long. "No-brain" philosophers cheerfully wave off all these problems as "easy." Consciousness stands alone as uniquely "hard." You can tell just by looking. Little do they know.

Later in his life, my dad wrote a weekly column called *Orchard Run*, printed in small-town newspapers up and down the Okanagan Valley. The expression "orchard run" refers to bulk fruit as it is shipped from the orchard, before it's prettied up for the supermarket and all the misshapen fruit is not yet culled out. His title allowed him the freedom to write in a homespun way about sensitive and complicated matters, especially concerning land use. Thus did he broach the long-term effects of logging and pesticides and the extermination of cougars. He wrote deftly about the predictable damage to a fragile ecology if the serpentine Okanagan River were dredged and dammed, and why the spawning salmon would probably never return.

Although my dad's *Orchard Run* columns were widely read, smarmy bureaucrats rode roughshod over the lived know-how of the Okanagan locals. Our bounteous river was reshaped into a lifeless canal, and its salmon never did return. Still, some sixty years later, plucky locals furtively released salmon fry from a fish farm into the canal and built fish ladders to allow the salmon to scale the dams. Some fry did find their way downstream to the Pacific Ocean, and four years later, a few salmon fought their way back upstream and searched for spawning grounds. As my father had broadly predicted in *Orchard Run*, nature as well as common sense will normally thrive, if you give them half a chance.

Grant Shreve

Writer, Scholar, Critic

Inspired Embarrassments: On Rough Drafts

This sentence—the one you're reading now—is not how this essay was going to start. Earlier drafts began otherwise: a historical narrative, a close reading of a literary passage, a ripped-from-the-headlines story. All tried and abandoned. None felt quite right.

If pressed, I could offer an explanation as to why I chose to begin so self-reflexively: the desire to surprise you—reader—through an act of apparent first-person disclosure. Truthfully, though, I'm not sure I can say with confidence why *this* and not *that*. Nor can I say whether this decision (or any other) was, ultimately, the right call. You won't be able to say, either. All the alternative paths this essay could have taken are shuttered. The false starts, dead ends, and abandoned sentences (in other words, the thousands upon thousands of accumulated keystrokes that led to what you're reading now) are buried on a hard drive. You probably aren't interested in reading them; I wouldn't be keen to share them.

That's more or less the natural order of things. Rough drafts are meant to be suppressed, hidden from view, tucked away in a literal or digital folder somewhere. They are the jetsam of writing, heaved overboard as soon as they've served their purpose. They are not *products*, but the ephemeral artifacts of *process*.

Or so we are conditioned to think. Yet drafts can never be just process, can they? They have heft and materiality. They are carefully crafted and labored over, and even shared with select audiences: that angelic host of peers, friends, teachers, and partners who suffer them and provide notes. Drafts, in short, straddle process and product, conception and completion. They are a liminal form, and that liminality evokes complex feelings, not always positive.

I, for instance, am among those writers who associate drafting primarily with shame. That is, I experience my own drafts less as verdant fields of generative potential and more as minefields of imminent

DOI: 10.4324/9781003516118-10

mortification. Whatever the genre—essay, speech, tweet and even the occasional email—the act of putting pen to paper (or finger to keyboard) usually fills me with dread at the prospect of confronting those first, halting sentence fragments that will rise like gas bubbles from my psyche as thought begins its search for shape. I see, then, glaringly, the weakness of my expression and the shallowness of my thinking. I start to imagine the reaction of future readers and picture them wincing at each misused word, sighing at each regurgitated idea or just looking generally baffled at the incoherence of the whole thing. Cue the anticipatory shame and embarrassment.

I am not alone in these feelings. Edgar Allan Poe was convinced that most writers "would positively shudder at letting the public take a peep behind the scenes, at the elaborate and vacillating crudities of thought." The literary critic D.A. Miller, in a study of Jane Austen's style, winced at what he called "the shame of the uncorrected," a feeling he identified as being acutely present in himself as well as Austen. Avoiding that shame (even posthumously) may be one reason so many authors arrange for the annihilation of their unfinished work, whether by incineration, shredding, or having their drafts—as the late fantasy writer Terry Pratchett requested—"put in the middle of the road and for a steamroller to steamroll over them all."

The obliteration of drafts is, however, almost always a loss. Notwithstanding those feelings of authorial shame, drafts can be a delight to experience for readers. They can enhance our appreciation of the work of others and demystify the labor of writing. Reading a draft, one gets to witness that moment, or, rather, series of moments, when ideas and stories previously suspended in the vacuum of a mind finally hit oxygen and touch solid ground.

Beginning in the 1970s, a cohort of textual scholars in France began reconceptualizing manuscript drafts as aesthetic objects worthy of critical attention and study. "Genetic criticism," as it came to be known, originated from a growing conviction that literary texts should be thought of not as hermetically sealed objects whose published form comprises the entirety of the text, but as the aggregate of all the drafts, outlines and notes (or pre-texts) that preceded it. In the words of genetic critic Pierre de Biasi, these pre-texts "constitute the very universe of *composition.*"

Few authors' oeuvres exemplify that claim more literally than that of the African American novelist Ralph Ellison, whose drafts taught me to love—and how to love—works-in-progress.

After publishing his 1952 debut novel, *Invisible Man*, to international acclaim, Ellison spent the next four decades (until his death in 1994) working on a follow-up. It was to be an American epic about the adopted (and racially ambiguous) son of a Black preacher who grows up to become a race-baiting United States senator subsequently assassinated by his own son on the floor of the Senate chamber. Ellison never finished it.

Housed in the Library of Congress, Ellison's drafts are voluminous, spanning tectonic social movements, multiple presidencies and several technological revolutions (evidenced by the fact that his earliest drafts were composed on a typewriter, and his final ones on a computer using the early word processing software WordStar). To read them is to experience an author's evolving relationship to his own drafts.

In the early years of his compositional saga, Ellison made significant progress on wresting his sweeping ideas about the contradictions and latent possibilities of American democracy into narrative form. But whether due to the ambition of the project, the pressure of living up to his debut, or the many private setbacks (including one house fire), he could never ultimately bring this work to a satisfactory close.

This was obviously anguishing for him. Yet, by the 1980s and '90s, something seemed to have changed in Ellison's relationship to the novel-in-progress. His late drafts are longer and more exploratory than anything he wrote in the decades prior. Devoid of virtually any dramatic tension or narrative propulsion, they meander and digress for hundreds of pages as characters indulge in lengthy meditations, dialogues and performances. They are, by turns, fascinating—representing some of the best writing of Ellison's career—and very boring. But that monotony is integral to their aesthetic. Reading these drafts feels like experiencing a mind allowing itself to roam through its own imaginative universe, free from the shame of incompletion or error and unburdened by an urgency to get somewhere. Ellison seems to have discovered that drafting and revising could be an activity without end, or even an end in itself. Long after it must have become clear to him that the novel would never be published in his lifetime, he kept writing.

This is not, however, to say these manuscripts are comfortable in their unfinishedness. They are laced with sadness, obstinacy and even a certain nostalgia. Written at the close of the twentieth century but set in the months and years before the U.S. Supreme Court's decision in *Brown v. Board of Education*, they feel yoked to an America that had long ceased to exist. The drafts are willfully belated, past their time. They are late in the sense that Edward Said describes, suffused with "the increasing sense of apartness and exile and anachronism."

But this belatedness is essential to the drafts' beauty and their difficulty. During one late draft sequence that takes place in a quasi-mythical Oklahoma nightclub called the Wind Cave, an audience member yells at the evening's chief entertainer, the storyteller Cliofus, to hurry up and stop wasting time. Cliofus responds with a line that could serve as a reflection on Ellison's novel and, indeed, the act of drafting itself: "Now just what the hell do words care about *time?*"

Words don't care about time, and neither do drafts. All too frequently, they defy the constraints of time, whether due to their sheer length or the delays in their completion. Their excesses and protractions upend the order and legibility toward which writing aspires. They overreach and stumble. In the process, they disclose all the tics, crutches, bad habits and "crudities of thought" of their all-too-fallible authors. As so many of us know, that can be shameful.

It can also be propulsive. One's literary weaknesses are (perhaps even ought to be) an invitation to keep probing, revising and producing. For writers and their readers alike, drafts are dense, wild thickets of thought and expression, always growing in new and surprising directions. The nineteenth-century critic Charles Lamb once complained of drafts that "the text never seems determinate. Print settles it." True enough, we might reply, but there are great pleasures and discoveries to be found in the still unsettled—embarrassing as it so often is.

Beverly J. Stoute

Psychoanalyst, Educator, Servant Leader

Revolution in the Mind

I took a deep breath standing at the ballroom lectern in the Hotel Saint Regis Detroit, the same city where, on June 23, 1963, Dr. Martin Luther King, Jr. first publicly spoke the words, "I have a dream."

During this sound check for my talk tomorrow, someone mentioned that Dr. King once spoke at that podium. An intense rush of emotion came over me: I was in the presence of ancestors.

Later, I returned to my hotel room to rework the introduction. This obsession to infuse words with emotion is my liability and my signature—a challenge every time I write or speak. I question myself. Can I do it? Am I living up to the legacy? I learned the basics of writing in school, but the drive to write and rewrite, the essence of being a writer, the urgent obsession to communicate the power of emotion, I learned from my father.

My father was a pioneering Black psychoanalyst, Quaker and civil rights activist. Growing up in a community-oriented family in New York, I was surrounded by physicians and leaders who shaped my sense of what a servant leader and Black intellectual should be. Childhood memories of my parents' dinner parties featured trailblazing civil rights activists whose scintillating debates fascinated and intrigued me. The question that was always asked: "What are you doing in the Movement today?" These dinners, the community organizing I witnessed and my father's leadership shaped my development as a writer and person.

A brilliant thinker and demanding teacher, my father spoke and wrote in five languages with power and beauty. He thought with quickness and razor-sharp wit. He taught me that writing requires vision, voice and perspective and attention to the audience. The right word carries meaning, the right argument persuades and the right nuance of feeling moves. Writing can express what we feel, and it moves others to feel, bringing people together.

DOI: 10.4324/9781003516118-11

My father had me read, study and memorize the work of great writers. The volumes on our bookshelves fascinated me. At the age of ten I selected a book from the collection of green volumes with gold lettering on the shelf in our living room. As I read the title, *A Tale of Two Cities*, and read Dickens's words, I was captivated. How did he take the pain of poverty and marginalization and infuse it with such beauty?

How did Charles Dickens write? ("It was the best of times, it was the worst of times . . . it was the epoch of belief, it was the epoch of incredulity . . . ")

How did Frederick Douglass write? ("What, to the American slave, is your 4th of July? . . . a day that reveals to him, more than all other days in the year, the gross injustice and cruelty to which he is the constant victim.")

How did James Baldwin write? ("If one is continually surviving the worst that life can bring, one eventually ceases to be controlled by a fear of what life can bring . . . ")

How did Dr. Martin Luther King, Jr. write? ("I have a dream this afternoon!")

My father fought racism with action and with his mind. He wrote to W.E.B. DuBois and asked him to join the demonstration when a Black professor at the University of Wisconsin was refused service at the faculty club. He typed the telegram message to First Lady Eleanor Roosevelt inviting her to attend a rally to fight segregation in sports. He typed the letter—in French—to President Kwame Nkrumah, and the leader of every other African nation, asking them to join an effort after independence to create a University of Africa and educate the next generation in anticolonial discourse. He corresponded with so many advocates who demonstrated for civil rights and education. After his death, I found the files of letters cleaning out his office and recognized the characteristic typeface of that old Royal typewriter he used to type every paper and letter. His Royal typewriter still sits dust-laden on my shelf as a symbol, a throughline of history, reminding me how my father waged revolution with words.

My father never seemed at a loss for words, especially when combating racist ideas. He taught me to talk to anyone about difficult topics with calm, compassion and the right words. He demanded specificity and concision, particularly when punctuating with emotion. He taught me that every essay should end with a philosophical statement of one's purpose in the world and create revolution in the mind.

As a child clinician, I reflect on how learning to write with my father was a form of play with words and ideas. He introduced me to history, philosophy, religion, politics and psychoanalysis, preparing me for battles he knew I would face. Knowledge, the precision of communication and achieving excellence, he taught me, would give me power. These lessons in warriorhood were a protective act of love, teaching me to fight racism with intellect and words.

Much later in my life I came to understand the throughline of his deep pain. Born in 1907, immigrating to the United States at the age of seventeen from the Caribbean, my outspoken father faced the obstacles of racial discrimination at every turn. He was kicked out of NYU for demonstrating against Jim Crow segregation in collegiate athletics, and later rejected from many medical schools because a Black activist was too much of a risk. He left to study at the Sorbonne when a Missouri-born professor blocked his PhD dissertation on implicit bias, a subject not yet in vogue in 1950.

France offered him, like so many Black thought leaders of his era, refuge from American racism as well as a new intellectual home. He finished four theses in French and completed the equivalent degree of a PhD, Docteur de l'Université en Sorbonne. Trying to become a Black psychoanalyst with a foreign degree at a time when there were none was considered near impossible, but not to him.

At eight, I told my parents I wanted to help kids so they wouldn't become adults with problems. I was curious about human behavior and driven by a desire to understand racism, a term my parents used to explain why my teachers at first would assume I was not smart.

When, as a child, I naively decided I wanted to be a psychoanalyst like him, his joy was stirred, and also his fear. He knew the obstacles I would face, and worked to strengthen me for the competitive white academic spaces I would traverse. His lessons in precision and emotional expression seemed, at times, tough and exacting, and still make me obsessionally precise, but these were lessons in warriorhood; for Black parents, lessons in warriorhood are necessary to a child's survival.

My father taught me: not just history, Black history. Not just great writers, Black writers. Not just leaders, Black leaders. Richard Wright, James Baldwin, Toni Morrison, Maya Angelou, W.E.B. DuBois, Alex Haley, Frederick Douglass, Paul Laurence Dunbar, Claude McKay, Langston Hughes, Ralph Ellison, Dr. Martin Luther King, Jr., Malcolm X, to name just a few. The writers he insisted I read connected me to a legacy of ancestral writers. After all, there is the African proverb: "If we stand tall it is because we stand on the shoulders of many ancestors."

When I write I am mobilizing pain, sacrifice and rage in a positive way; I am engaging in an act of resistance, a continuation of a fight that my ancestors and my father waged. If I, as a writer, find just the right words to make some piece of myself known, then I share the pains of injustice with you, my reader. You and I become "we," just as I became "we" with those who wrote before me. As I write, I am with my father;

we are still trying to make an incomprehensible world comprehensible. Am I, I ask, bringing you into what I feel?

When I write, I hope for moments of connection. Can I inspire *you* to question the injustices and inequities of our world? Can you share in the pain of what I know? Can we become known to each other if I elicit emotional resonance with these words? When writing, I feel a sense of urgency to communicate, and to connect to you as my imagined audience. There is the possibility of a "we" with mutual compassion and empathy in the world—if only I find the right words.

Natasha Trethewey

Poet, Memoirist, Professor

Articulation

A poem

—After Miguel Cabrera's portrait of Saint Gertrude, 1763

In the legend, Saint Gertrude is called to write
after seeing, in a vision, the sacred heart of Christ.

Cabrera paints her among the instruments
of her faith: quill, inkwell, an open book,

rings on her fingers like Christ's many wounds—
the heart emblazoned on her chest, the holy

infant nestled there as if sunk deep in a wound.
Against the dark backdrop, her face is a wafer

of light. How not to see, in the saint's image,
my mother's last portrait: the dark backdrop,

her dress black as a habit, the bright edge
of her afro ringing her face with light? And how

not to recall her many wounds: ring finger
shattered, her ex-husband's bullet finding

her temple, lodging where her last thought lodged?
Three weeks gone, my mother came to me

in a dream, her body whole again but for
one perfect wound, the singular articulation

DOI: 10.4324/9781003516118-12

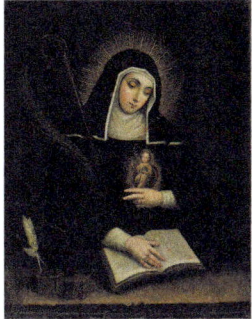

Figure 1.1 Permissions Line: *Saint Gertrude (Santa Gertrudis)*, 1763, Miguel Cabrera. Oil on canvas, 43 1/2 × 34 3/4 in. Dallas Museum of Art, gift of Laura and Daniel D. Boeckman in honor of Dr. William Rudolph, 2006.37

of all of them: a hole, center of her forehead,
the size of a wafer—light pouring from it.

How, then, could I not answer her life
with mine, she who saved me with hers?

And how could I not—bathed in the light
of her wound—find my calling there?

Permissions Line: "Articulation" from *Monument: Poems New and Selected* by Natasha Trethewey. Copyright © 2018 by Natasha Trethewey. Used by permission of HarperCollins Publishers.

Julius W. Hobson, JR.

Lobbyist, Adjunct Professor

Growing up in a glass house with one or more "famous" parents is not what it's cracked up to be.

I am an African American native of Washington, D.C., and largely the product of a civil rights family. Most recognize me as the son of Julius W. Hobson, Sr., a major civil rights leader in the District of Columbia. Through his meetings in our basement, I met several prominent leaders, including Kwame Ture (Stokely Carmichael). My father was the founder of the D.C. Statehood Party, a member of the first elected Board of Education and a member of the first elected City Council. For a good portion of my life, I was criticized for not being like my father.

My father was also seen as a radical who frightened folks, especially some Black folks. Some people hated him. In the first quarter of 10th grade, I was flunked in biology and geometry because the teachers hated him—and said so.

Because I was my father's son, the FBI opened a file on me when I was fourteen (my sister is eight years younger than I am and missed out on her own file). I know this because I have read it.

Years later, George Washington University turned me down three times, first as an undergraduate. I matriculated instead at Howard University. There, one professor returned my mid-term exam on the last day of class marked with an "F." He singled me out as the dumbest person in the class. It had been an open-book exam; I happened to use a book he had not read.

For four years during the Vietnam era, I was a member of the Army ROTC at Howard. I achieved outstanding military student status, yet I was the only member of my class whose loyalty was interrogated by military intelligence. In the end, the Army sent me a letter saying they did not need me.

In short, growing up Black, growing up as Julius Hobson, Jr., had extra challenges—still does.

When I was chair of the board of D.C. General Hospital—the public hospital in the city largely serving poor and working-class African

DOI: 10.4324/9781003516118-13

Americans—I held a full day all-employee meeting to discuss the coming closure of the hospital. As I tried to help employees understand what was about to happen, a man stood up and said loudly, "Your father must be turning over in his grave because you are nothing like him!"

My response to that has always been: "Have you ever met my mother?"

My mother, Carol Joy Hobson Smith, had a profound effect on people. She was a career federal government civil servant; a deeply religious person, her civil rights activities emanated from her church activities. Through her church activities, I met Rev. Andrew Young, Jr. Civil rights lawyer and professor Derrick Bell was also a member of the church before moving to Boston to teach at Harvard Law School. Kwame Ture gravitated to my mother because he absolutely loved her cooking. When I last saw him on Howard University's campus, his first words were questions about how my mother was doing. Very few knew of my mother and her influence.

My mother was my personal tutor for as long as I can remember. Through elementary school she covered every subject. She was a perfectionist who knew the world I was entering. My mother led by example. She became the first executive director of the first Department of Education advisory committee on Black higher education and Black colleges and universities. By the end of her career, she had mentored dozens of up-and-coming Black Federal government civil servants. Through work and retirement, until dementia limited her capacity during the last year of her long life, she would school anyone on their writing or speech.

When George Washington University again turned me down, this time for graduate school, they agreed I could take courses, but attached the proviso that I must take the Graduate Record Exam (GRE)—an exam not required of other applicants—and that, after twelve course hours, I have a 3.0 GPA. Only after eighteen hours was I granted full admission. I have a photograph taken at graduation of me with the dean and department chair who had signed the letter enumerating the extra work that would be required for my admission. The photograph was taken because my mother insisted. Ironically, in 2020, I was honored as a distinguished graduate.

In my first job as a government relations professional, I represented Howard University. At the time I was hired, there were only a handful of Black professional lobbyists—and I had no mentor. To compensate, I read everything I could get my hands on. Since then, I have built a personal library of over 3,000 nonfiction books and counting. I have had to teach myself in the same manner and with the same rigor with which my mother taught me.

In the public policy process, as in politics, words matter. How public policy is rhetorically presented can make the difference between public acceptance or opposition. In my 50 years in the public policy business, I have worn many hats. In the United States Senate, I was the professional on Senator Charles Robb's (D-VA) staff responsible for appropriations, the budget, financial services and taxes. Every year, an association came to our office to press their concerns. Each year for four years, they would ask me how I had come to work for the Senator. And every year, they asked the Senator who in the office they should talk to. To his credit, Robb would point to me. My mother's insistence that I write and speak precisely played an important part in Robb's respect for me and my work. Those skills of communication are part of my reputation.

As an adjunct professor at George Washington University's Graduate School of Political Management since 1994, I have been teaching the course on lobbying. In the first years, before there was general access to the internet, many students on the first night of class looked shocked that their professor was Black.

In those early years, some students would challenge my knowledge. One, who turned in all his assignments late, did so in a formal appeal of the grade he earned. I developed a reputation as the toughest grader in the school. Thanks to my mother, I was, and am, demanding about both the grammar and substance of my students' assignments. Grammar and diction create meaning and intent. They make things better understood and they make things happen; they create respect.

For over eight years, I have also taught "Legislative Writing and Research." I find this the most exciting course to teach. My students write press releases, decision memoranda, position papers, op-eds, Congressional floor statements, legislative text summaries and Congressional witness testimony.

I teach that when reading or drafting legislation, the "action" word chosen makes a big difference. "May" means the executive branch has discretion; "shall" forces action. Removing a colon and inserting a semicolon can change a bill substantially. In the public arena, I discovered that by using language precisely I could affect public policy. In teaching legislative writing, I pass on what I learned growing up: punctuation matters, words matter.

The late professional basketball player Bill Russell was known for his strong defense on the court. In an interview, he was asked his secret. Russell responded, saying, "I establish position." That resonates. It applies to my life—and to work in the public policy arena as well. You "establish position" by becoming a walking library of the regulatory and legislative process and of the issues. You then must communicate what you know with words that can be readily understood.

Shortly after changing his name from Cassius Clay to Muhammad Ali, Ali fought Ernie Terrell. In a pre-fight gathering, Terrell refused to call Ali by his new name, and insisted on calling him Cassius Clay. As a freshman at Howard University, on February 6, 1967, I recall listening on the radio to their fight. Ali hit Terrell unmercifully for fifteen rounds and could have knocked him out in any of those rounds. After each punch, Ali yelled "What's my name?"

Since then, I have been a member of the "call me by the name I have chosen" fan club. Professor. Public Policy Lobbyist. Writer. Son of Julius and Carol. Brother. Husband. Father. Grandfather.

Orlando Patterson

Professor, Public Intellectual

The Dresswriter

My motivation to write, what drives me and my initial inspiration all come from different sources. I was *motivated* by the urge to understand the bleakness of my early social environment and the immediacy of my brutal slave past. I grew up in one of the dreariest and most impoverished parts of colonial Jamaica. May Pen was a market town in the parched middle of the island, surrounded by sugar plantations where ragged, barefooted canecutters still toiled as their ancestors had done for centuries under the hideous exploitation of British slaveholders. Those who escaped the cruel fields worked from dawn to dusk on hopelessly small, gravelly grounds from which they scratched yam heads and withered beans in a hand-to-mouth existence.

I went to school with their children, who came late each morning, their bare feet cracked from the miles of hot marl roads they had to walk and run on, the swollen lesions of itching jiggers exposed between their toes. Hungry and already too tired to learn, the whippings by the sadistic pupil teachers for being late made sure they didn't. They were absent from our large initial classes of seventy or more students early, first on Thursdays and Fridays to help on the farms and prepare for market, then, by the age of ten, were nearly all gone for good. This made for smaller classes and, for me and those other kids who stayed in school, slightly better teaching. But it was an uneasy, slightly guilty comfort. Even as a child I felt that there was something wrong about their absence. I knew that I was no more intelligent than several of them who were now destined for the cane fields and barren farms. I became more and more aware of the past that haunted every aspect of life, especially the Indian "coolie" laborers who had been brought into the island after slavery to replace the slaves who fled the plantations for the emerging peasantry. Something was wrong, I kept thinking, and the growing desire to know more, to feel less unease about the country that the emerging nationalist movement was calling "homeland" motivated me to write.

DOI: 10.4324/9781003516118-14

One of my earliest short stories, published in the Sunday literary page of the island's leading newspaper, *The Daily Gleaner*, was about a cane field set on fire by disgruntled workers. Another mourned the fate of a teenager of my age who had gone to England with the Windrush migration, only to find herself trafficked in the British sex trade. That early story got me into serious trouble with the prudish headmaster of my Anglican grammar school, who, threatening suspension, wanted to know what a choirboy had to do with the brothels of the mother country. Sir, I protested innocently, I've never left the island.

I was *driven* to write by the linguistic vagaries and contradictions of my early colonial education. My first language was Creole, the vernacular that had emerged from the days of slavery out of the syncretism of English and West African languages. It was the language of home, of play and ordinary interactions. At school, though, we were commanded to speak the King's—and later Queen's—English, and the poorer students, who spoke only Creole, were whipped for failing to learn it, another reason for their early departure. My mother had already taught me the basics of "proper" English by reading to me from a book of stories based on Shakespeare's plays, then, when I learned to read with some fluency, turned the tables on me by insisting that I read the *Daily Gleaner* to her each day after school as she worked at her dressmaking. At first, I was only decoding, since the newspaper's vocabulary and the political stories she directed me to read were unintelligible. But I slowly came to understand the meaning of the words and by the age of eight or nine was quite knowledgeable about the nation's politics. It also helped that I had to accompany her on her early morning canvassing for the People's National Party whose great nationalist leader—Norman Manley, a Rhodes Scholar and Queen's Counsel—she cherished as a model for what she wanted her son to become.

At school, we were taught to read and write "properly" from the *Royal Readers*, a series of imperial textbooks for British children with illustrated moral prose pieces, poems and outlines of British History, propagated throughout the schools of the empire. After dictations, precis and recitations on the beauty of the British landscape, and the derring-dos of great British heroes—among them slave mongers, privateers and other sanctified scoundrels—we were asked to write short essays on "our" ancestors and glorious island, the one, that is, in the North Atlantic with its "host of golden daffodils." It was actually quite a challenge to the imagination of a Jamaican child to write about "a winter's day" and, contrary to post-colonial outrage, drove one to think as a writer should, conceiving worlds unknown. But even more challenging were the essay topics, which the teachers wickedly favored, on "a summer's day." They knew what they were doing. Asking a child in a sweltering tropical island to write about a summer's day, especially with the British assumption that it was to be wished for, is like asking a fish in a muddy pond to write about water. Imagining the obvious is far more difficult than conjuring what's different. Those exercises drove me early to some of the subtler demands of writing—but only after several whacks across my back from those pupil-teachers.

It was, however, my mother's dressmaking that *inspired* me most to write. She was a mistress of her craft which, during my childhood in the middle of the last century, was the livelihood of thousands of working class Jamaican single mothers. I often helped her, not only by keeping her up to date on the news while she sewed, but by threading her needles, holding one end of a misaligned cut of fabric while she pulled to square it up and shopping for buttons and other trimmings. But what captivated me most about her work was her cutting of the dress parts from the cloth her customers brought. She had the rare talent of being able to cut out dresses without a pattern, which she never used. Her customers would turn up with their fabric and an image of the style of dress they wanted torn from the newspaper or a magazine. Sometimes they would sit and select one from the dog-eared set of women's magazines she kept, mainly one called *Seventeen*, an American lady's journal which, for some strange reason, Jamaican young women of mid-century seemed to favor.

I wrote down the measurements of her customers in a lined exercise book sitting by the dining table that also served as her cutting board. Most women at that time wore slips, so I didn't have to leave the room when they undressed. Occasionally, for those without slips, I would sit on our little front porch, and she would call them out: height, bust, shoulder, center back, waist, hips, sometimes around the knees and mid-calf for women who wanted the hobble, which was all the rage among Jamaican women when I was in my late singles. I loved doing that. It made me feel directly engaged in helping her make our living. In the same exercise book beneath the measurements, I also kept the cost of making each dress: the buttons, pipings, ribbons, braids and other trimmings which it was also my little job to buy, after matching carefully with clippings of the fabric, at the local Syrian dry-goods shop. I took matching seriously, paying no attention to the giggles of the shop clerks waiting on me, who marveled that a child, much less a boy, would be asked to do such a thing. Pipings were a challenge: never the same color, she always cautioned, but close. I learned much selecting buttons, which later I came to think were just like metaphors that bind and beautify.

What most intrigued me, and the lesson about how to do anything really important—especially writing—was the way my mother went about the cutting of her dresses. This always drew my attention, and I would often stop what I was doing to watch her as she did it. Her countenance seriously darkened, the cinnamon-toned brow deeply furrowed, which used to startle me when I was much younger. She became unusually quiet, and never hummed her favorite hymns as she did when sewing or doing other chores. Her hands moved swiftly as she cleared and cleaned the cutting table. She laid out the fabric, then carefully folded it, aligning the grainline by matching the selvages. Sometimes she would huff with annoyance if the shop had not cut the fabric straight, which she would fix, using the edges of the table to get a sharp angle, after which she would close her eyes, take a deep breath and, upon regaining her concentration, begin to measure up the material. Occasionally, on lighter-colored fabric, she used a tailor's chalk to mark the measurements, but she disliked chalk, finding it, she once told me, too mannish and persistent, especially with the more delicate fabrics, preferring instead to use tracings of thread, basting the markings loosely through the fabric, as she folded and unfolded it.

After marking the measurements, she stopped, leaned over the fabric, her arms stretched out at an angle on either side of it, and stared intently for several minutes, rehearsing every move, every cut she planned to make. For me, that was always the scariest and most wonderful part. I knew, as she did, that one mistake, one cut too long, or in the wrong direction, however small, could ruin everything. Instead of being paid, she would be paying for the damaged fabric, and maybe lose a customer. We might go hungry for a while. This rarely happened. With a deep breath she took up her scissors and began to cut. Once she started cutting, she never stopped until she was through. She cut swiftly, sure-handedly, sometimes using the scissors like a knife to cut long lengths, sometimes just snipping at the tips, and sometimes, for the longest cuts, if the fabric permitted, she would make what for me was always the most daring move: after a snip, she would lift the entire fabric up, hold it tightly on either side of the snip and rip it apart with a swift sweep of her arms until they were stretched far apart and the fabric fell like open curtain panels beside her. After cutting she took a deep, restorative breath and stared for a long time at the cut and pinned fabric, like a hunter staring at her kill. Then, she wrapped the fabric together and put it away. Rarely did she sew right after cutting. Instead, she went about some other task—cleaning our two small rooms, lighting the charcoal for our meal in the outdoor kitchen, sometimes showering in the old bathroom next to it.

To be sure, writing is far more forgiving than cutting dresses without a pattern. The dresses that writers fabricate are, as they might say in the dressmaker's trade, loose clothing with lots of ease, allowing for repeated editing. There was little ease in the hobble, and even less in the curved necklines, shawl collars and hourglass shapes of the New Look that my mother's clients had to have, whatever their shapes or sizes.

What I learned from this repeated display of concentrated craftswomanship sunk in deeply and was applied to most demanding things I've had to do, especially my writing. I've often read of other writers modeling their early work on those of established authors. I have never felt the urge to do that. The influence of others, as I'm sure occurred, had to be subconscious. Consciously, it became ingrained in me to work without another's pattern. Indeed, to always go against the grain, as a mentor of my adult years, David Riesman, once advised me. To prepare, to take the measure of the task, to think it through over and over, to begin only when truly ready and, once begun, not stop until what was planned was finished, was my method, starting with those earliest schoolboy essays in defiance of the *Royal Readers* and with dressmaking, where there was only one chance to edit when the customers came to fit.

2

Urges and Traumas

Ellen Pinsky and Michael Slevin

Louis Menand

Writer, Professor

Why Did I Write About Why I Write?

I believe that everything happens for a reason, and that the goal of non-fiction writing, which is the kind of writing I do, is to give the reason.

You do this by first ascertaining the facts of the matter. I'm a material-ist, and I like data; I don't believe in the Zeitgeist or the spirit of the age or magical thinking as an explanatory entity. I like information, verifiable facts. But the facts don't speak for themselves. The facts have to be fitted together, like the pieces of a puzzle, so that they make a picture or tell a story. The facts are out there; you can't mess with them. But the com-pleted picture is yours, something you create. That picture is the creative part of "creative nonfiction." It is not something you have found; it is something you have imagined based on the stuff you have found. You assemble the picture by applying to the facts whatever wisdom or insight or just feel for things you've managed to derive from life. It's your intui-tion that makes the facts sensible. I'm not sure whether this is something that can be taught. Maybe it is.

If you're a magazine writer, which I am, besides informing your read-ers, you also need to interest, entertain, and excite them. You want to keep the reader on the page. The definition of good writing is writing that it is harder to stop reading than to keep reading. *Every sentence* needs to interest, entertain, and hold out the promise of something unexpected. Great sentences are what it's all about, because people read one sen-tence at a time, and it's easy to change the channel. They just turn the page. Your piece is competing with every other piece in the magazine, not to mention every screen within reach, for someone's attention.

Reading a poem or a piece of fiction, you anticipate a surprise—a twist, a reveal, a frisson. In nonfiction writing, the surprise is a novel take, what is called, in the magazine business, the "hook." The hook is unique. It's what makes your piece on a subject that everyone else is also cover-ing distinctive—smarter, more moving, more exciting, more fun. Looking out for, or enjoying, the hook is what keeps the reader on the page.

DOI: 10.4324/9781003516118-16

I've written hundreds of pieces of this description. Some are eight hundred words long and some are eight thousand words long, but all of them are meant to be read in one sitting and all of them have the same formal structure: here are the facts, and here is the picture they make. I have written editorials, but I don't usually write one-sided pieces, or pieces that are meant to provoke. I want everyone to agree with me (although, sadly, they don't). My job is to help people think, not to tell people what to think. Some of my pieces work better than others, but I would say that ninety percent of the time, I'm happy with what I wrote. That's what makes it possible for me to write again, because writing, let's face it, is work.

If everything happens for a reason, then what is the reason I write? And why do I write the kind of pieces I do? The fact that I have been doing this at a more or less regular rate of production for forty years suggests that the desire to make things out of words—to create verbal artifacts, to give it a grander name—is innate. It's something I wake up with every day. It's compulsive in the same degree that stamp-collecting or marathon training is compulsive. This is what I am engineered to do. (I can do other things as well!)

It's true that I get money and career advancement by writing. Like any writer, at least any magazine writer, I want people to like what I write, and the more people who like it, the better, because, in the industry, readership is the name of the game. I never write except for publication. Otherwise, it's like performing a comedy routine just for yourself. You need someone else to laugh. In the end, though, having an audience and getting paid is not why I do it. I could write a lot less. The pleasure it gives me to make pieces is worth more to me than the pleasure my pieces give to others—as long as others reads it.

This is one subject—why I write—that I'm not sure I can give a reason for. It may be that I don't really want to know what drives this thing in me, or how the mechanism works. There is something, I don't want to say magical, but ineffable about it. I can try to describe what it feels like, though. That can't hurt.

I suspect that everyone who is a writer has had some intense experience with reading. That's kind of how you know you want to write. When I was little, I tried to read the grown-up books my parents owned, but I never got far in them. My first passion was the Hardy Boys mysteries. I was a Hardy Boys binge reader. I checked the books out of the town library and read them in bed at night. The third book in the Hardy Boys series is *The Secret of the Old Mill*. Frank and Joe, boy detectives, are on the trail of a band of counterfeiters who have set up their counterfeiting operation in an abandoned mill. One night, Frank and Joe sneak into the attic of the mill, and they watch, through a crack in the floorboards, the counterfeiters at work below. Lying in my bed, as I read this chapter, my heart started pounding. I was *there* with Frank and Joe, looking through the crack, holding my breath so I wouldn't make a sound that might let the counterfeiters know they were being spied on.

Somehow, this inert string of marks on a page was creating not just words I recognized from speech, but sensations. The marks were literally making my pulse race. At some subconscious level, I thought: *I want to do this*. I want to put letters on a page that will cause people's hearts to pound, cause people's skin to crawl, cause people's minds to change.

I wrote my first poem when I was fourteen. It was about the Battle of Thermopylae. I have no idea what inspired me to compose verses on that topic, but I do remember, even now, that the act of composition was absorbing. I can remember where I was sitting in the school library when I finished it. Writing a poem is like writing anything but more so: a matter of getting the right words in the right order. What appealed to me in that process was that you are completely in charge. It's *your* words in *your* order. You have absolute power to determine whether a word goes in or comes out. There is no appeal. Not a lot of life is like that.

I switched to lyric poetry, poems intended to evoke a mood or an attitude. I wrote poetry in high school and all through college. I'm being honest, not modest, when I say that the poems I wrote in school were pretty bad, even by schoolboy standards. I think this was because, verbal dexterity aside, I had nothing particular to say. I also don't like to write about myself. I don't really like writing this. It just gave me pleasure back then to make a poem. I was writing for the sake of writing.

After I graduated from college, I had to write critical papers. And I discovered, a little to my surprise, that writing non-fiction prose gave me exactly the same pleasure I had writing poems. It was a matter of putting the right words in the right order; I was in charge; the process was absorbing. Writing nonfiction also gave me something to write about that was independent of my feelings and personal experiences. Yet I found that I could express myself much more fully and honestly in impersonal nonfiction than I ever could in poetry. The sensibility producing the words was *me*. Or, more precisely, the me I want to be.

Good writing gives the impression of being effortless, but it rarely is. If the writer is not slaving over it, some editor probably is. For me, writing a piece, or a book chapter, which has the same format, demands a lot of preparation, a lot of fact finding. I need to get as much information in my head as I can. I never jot down ideas or make an outline. I just prepare until I think I've got it. I have an idea about how I want readers to experience the piece and, usually, about how it will end, and then I write a sentence. When I'm happy with that sentence, I write another sentence. When I write the last sentence, the piece is done. I don't go back.

Where do the sentences come from? The hardest part is the first sentence or two. They determine the tone and scale of the piece. I see that to fulfill their promise, I will need to cover X amount of material and to aim for Y effect. To get those first sentences, I need to get in touch with (to use a bad metaphor) my voice.

My writing voice is not the everyday me. It's some inner me. I think of it as "Luke," which is the nickname my parents gave me and is still the name I'm called by. (I don't identify as Louis. It's a byline. The reasoning for that is complicated and possibly unsound.) Luke has a certain way of "speaking," a certain take on things, a certain level of insight that the everyday in-person me does not have, or not as coherently. It can take a while, sometimes two or three days, for this voice to be heard. But once I hear it, I can begin.

When I have the facts, I don't begin writing immediately. I wait a day or two. I believe (I think most people know this experience) that the brain organizes information and solves problems subconsciously. It's the "sleep on it" phenomenon. The debris of research has to settle for a story to emerge. Luke is the name for whatever in my head it is that knows the story. Luke tells the story to me. I just write it down.

Once Luke emerges, the writing becomes (sort of) fun. Fun in the way being on stage is fun. I'm playing a character, and the character is myself. I would say, maybe, my best self—infinitely subtle, infinitely tolerant, infinitely disillusioned but never cynical. It could be that I write because I can "be" the person I think I am, or want to be, more fully on the page than I can in life. I can't fix the errors and bad choices I make every day, but I can fix errors and bad choices on the page. Writing is a way for me to edit myself, a way for me to be a better person.

Now I see that I have written a piece that has no facts, has no hook, and is completely about me. Why did I do that?

Louise Glück

Poet

It seems to me that I have wanted to write for the whole of my life. The intensity of this insistence, despite its implausibility, suggests an emotional, rather than literal, accuracy. I think my life didn't seem *my* life until I started to write.

I came from a family of talkers. But talk, in my house, was not conversation. Talk was holding forth. Prevailing. Having the last word. Only one person could do it at a time, which meant there was constant barging in and interruption, as impatience to speak grew more feverish and more relentless. Everybody wanted to talk. Nobody wanted to listen. In this, I was exactly like my mother and father and sister, though we had, each of us, a distinctive style. More and more the sentences I had in my head were like the sentences I loved in books: they began in one way and ended somewhere you had never imagined, though at each turn idea seemed to follow idea perfectly naturally. The surprise at the end, as the thought completed itself, seemed wildly exciting: the whole of the sentence needed to be re-experienced in this light; waves of unexpected revelations and insights resulted. Paradox. But an interrupted paradox is not simply edited. It is fundamentally changed, sometimes into the orderly, reasonable opposite it seemed destined to be. Because I never got to finish what I intended to say, response (on the rare occasions when it occurred) never seemed a response to my thought, but rather to the simplified idea it had become.

I came to have a sense that the self I was in the world, among other selves, was alternately precarious and invisible. I did not think speech was a good conduit to the self, or expression of it, because in my childhood it was not. The page was different. Here my voice had a stability and immutability, qualities I passionately craved and never remotely approached in my social interactions. How could I? Stability and immutability are not characteristics of the spoken word.

I learned to read at a very early age. And I began writing at the same time. My father also wrote. He wrote witty rhymed verses, doggerel;

DOI: 10.4324/9781003516118-17

I had the sound of doggerel in my head as far back as memory goes. I knew how rhyme worked. I heard the way rhythmic patterns conferred a strange sense of wholeness and inevitability. I began to write my own versions of this sort of poem, little bleak existential ditties, using the vocabulary available to me at, say, five years old:

> If kittycats liked roastbeef bones
> And doggies sipped up milk;
> If elephants walked around the town
> All dressed in purest silk;
> If robins went out coasting,
> They slid down, crying whee,
> If all this happened to be true
> Then where would people be?

My sister and I were also writing books. My father was our scribe. We made up stories and he wrote them down on pieces of paper folded to make books; afterward, when the writing had been completed, my sister and I drew illustrations in the large spaces left for them. None of these books still exist, to my knowledge, but I remember how they looked. I remember the joy of making things up; I remember the absorption, the world falling away.

Making up stories, making up anything, seemed to me the most involving and wonderful activity I could possibly imagine. And the story seemed, in some way, more important than anything in the world, I suppose because it was not subject to change. I imagine people believe in God for the same reason.

In the poems I was writing then, the pleasures of doggerel united with the wild happiness of inventing something that would have a separate existence, more convincing and more durable than my unreliable human existence. Those poems *were* me; they represented or embodied me. But, at the same time, they were not me; they were a thing apart that could be studied and adjusted and made perfect, as my actual self could not be. I was the writer; I was also the reader. The immersive creative act gave rise to analytic distance as the finished poem detached itself from its author. I had no control over the writing self, which seemed vulnerable to chance and whim, about which I had constant anxiety. But I had infinite control as a reader, a critic. Control and stamina and intense investment. Imperfect details and conventional perceptions tormented me; these problems I attempted to resolve, even in childhood. The process was called revision, I later learned, though this word seemed a little calm for an effort so protracted and often so hopeless.

Writing became almost immediately the form of communication that seemed to me most true and least fraught. Important conversations are routinely remembered differently. Of speech, an impression remains, which memory amplifies and distorts. No two people hearing the same remarks are likely to have identical memories of what was said. The exact words, certainly, will not be remembered. Whereas the written word can be remembered *only* exactly; if a written line is not repeated exactly, word for word, it is not being remembered, it is being paraphrased. The existing text will confirm this. In that text, words do not mutate or switch places. Meaning can be disputed, but the actual words survive argument and mutilation.

But with whom was I communicating? Unclear. In part with myself—I was learning what, or at least how, I thought. In part with strangers, my imagined ideal readers, most of whom were not yet born. In part with the future, a time when I would not exist to explain myself.

The things I wrote down so urgently were not fixed thoughts projected from my brain onto the page. What I considered thought was a kind of seeking, a mission. But it was very difficult. This was not writing as rhetoric or catharsis. This was writing as transformation (or this is what I wanted it to be). I wanted to turn experience, often disappointment or hurt, into an externalized form that, in its accuracy and beauty, would both separate me from the experience and redeem it. The need to write in this way was constant, but the ability to write at all came and went; often in my life it was gone for years. This was not something I could do anything about.

I had, in regard to making poems, no feeling of agency at all. Words and phrases came from nowhere; I rarely had any sense of what they meant or to what context they belonged. Nor could I access the source of these fragments. Whatever their source, I was either its victim (if I was hearing nothing) or its beneficiary. I felt, in childhood, like Joan of Arc in the story my father told my sister and me at bedtime, with the burning omitted. Joan, who heard voices and saved France. I heard voices, too. I heard pieces of phrases. But I did not have any idea what they were telling me.

I was exalted but also tormented. What I heard was suggestive, haunting, but unintelligible. In any case, I often heard nothing. But when I did hear I was possessed.

My task was to discover what the words meant. Who said them. Why. The method by which these investigations were conducted will be well known to psychoanalysts and analytic patients. The object, in fact, is not so different. In its most essential terms, the object is always to discover the self.

The method is free association. What I did in analysis imitated for me what I did as a writer. Analysis seemed a parallel search, with its constant re-examination of connections and transitions, the archetypal stories varied or not in each retelling; this tracking of thought was like writing, but with a crucial difference. Free association in writing, when writing is actually going on and not merely longed for, is euphoric; thought seems to move upward and skyward, the panorama widening, the material available to the gaze increasing as one rises farther away. Whereas in analysis, association spirals downward. Toward origins. Toward bedrock. Capitulation or recognition and later, sometimes, clarity. But not exaltation.

There is a second difference. In analytic association, the tool or the instrument is memory. Memory is examined, and also the juxtaposition of memories that are not sequential. Other journeys occur, but this, in my experience, is the central one. This is not what happens in the making of a poem. Memories may flicker here and there, but the associative leaps are almost exclusively related to language, and the shape of the poem is the shape made of the implications and atmospheres inherent in particular words or particular syntactical structures. So the process is in some essential way abstract, a kind of trailblazing that has no basis in lived event.

There remains a strange relation to the poems already written. Though they were written to create or affirm my existence, they did not, once they were finished, continue to do so. What they suggested, when I read them afterward, was that I had once existed and had thoughts; something that had been alive and specific was now silent or vanished. So the poems became a kind of chastisement, taunting reminders of what was not.

How different all this is, in its essence and outcome, from physical life. In the great physical events, extreme bodily pleasure and extreme bodily suffering, the self disappears completely or is lost. Either way, an involuntary act, unlike the struggle to be, to exist, that underlies the need to write.

I wrote a short book last summer, in prose, about a pair of twins living through their first year. One of them, despite being pre-verbal, is obsessed with the idea of the book she will one day write—is already writing in her head, though she has no words. Her name in my book is Marigold. Her sister, who is less driven, more gregarious, and easy to love, is Rose. And Marigold knows that she needs to write her book because she needs there to be something in the world "that stood for herself as Rose stood for Rose."

Permissions Line: DRIVEN TO WRITE contribution by Louise Glück. Copyright © Louise Glück Estate, March 2025, by permission of The Wylie Agency (UK) Limited.

Nazila Fathi

Writer, Journalist

The uninterrupted sound of the intercom jolts me out of bed. Shamsi summons Mom every morning at 5:00 AM for their walk. I imagine her, four-foot-six, with her finger on the buzzer until the elevator door opens and she sees Mom. That is when she lifts her finger and I can go back to sleep.

I am having breakfast when mom walks in with our weekly milk ration and she explains that Shamsi spotted the line after their walk. She pretended to organize the queue and then, in a moment of confusion, walked to the front and got milk for both of them. The neighbors are kind to her because they know about her husband. Once a deputy minister of health, he may, like so many others, face the firing squad any day. The revolutionaries jailed him for his ties to the previous regime. For five years, every Friday Shamsi visits him, thinking this would be their last encounter.

Later that day, I sit on a bench with a new girl watching the boys in the pool. On their olive-colored skin, the beads of water shine under the blistering sun. How I miss my gutsy friend who left for the United States. If she were here, we would just dive into the pool with all the layers of clothes that the revolutionaries make us wear to cover the curves of our bodies. We would ignore the persistent sound of the lifeguard's whistle eager to get us out of the pool. Instead, I would bury my face in the water as I did so many times, and swim, pushing forward in the heavy wet pants, knee-length coat and the t-shirt underneath. We would swim an entire exhilarating lap before running home and leaving a wet trail behind us.

"Watch out," the boys yell. Three of them run, and mid-air they hug their knees, making a big splash as they land in the water. We laugh and immediately feel cooler. We are not entitled to even these droplets of water for we should not be anywhere near half-naked boys. But pushing the boundaries makes us feel alive, especially at the age of fourteen.

DOI: 10.4324/9781003516118-18

Back home, I need to escape the reality of my life where I have no control over anything beyond my room. I shut the door and grab the third volume of *The Enchanted Soul* in Persian. My latest hero is Annette Riviere, the fictional character that French author Romain Rolland created during the storms of wartime in the early 1900s in Paris. Annette, the young protagonist, finds out after her father's death that she has a half-sister, Sylvie, a tailor who is into fashion and vies to live life to the fullest. The two women immediately develop a sisterly bond. Although they have very different characters, they complement and flow into each other's lives as their last name, meaning river in French, suggests.

But it is Annette who is extraordinary. She breaks up her wedding to a wealthy and educated young man that she loves. She believes he lacks culture, imagination and human relationships, and is no match for her with her yearning to grow and be free. "The union of two beings ought not to become a mutual enchainment. It should be a twofold blooming. I should like each, instead of being jealous of each other's free development, to be happy in assisting it," she believes. She goes on to give birth to his son out of wedlock. Her courage and strength seep into my mind and begin to shape my thinking about who I want to become.

I am safe with Annette. I prefer to be with her in Paris before the war than in the Islamic Republic of Iran during a war. So, I read through the night.

#

Annette leads the way and ushers me into the world of feminism with such force that I never leave for the rest of my life. But that is not all. She is an intellectual, an activist and a system of thoughts that helps me think about what happens around me—the violence, my friends and relatives fleeing the country, restrictions on my life as a girl and countless other issues that are beyond the comprehension of an adolescent. Her ideas resonate with me and enable me to think through events that I unconsciously distance myself from. "What a hard thing to witness, human civilization is based on a trembling base, continuing on a basis of the habit. Soon this tower is about to collapse." Her words carry weight—not the kind that crushes you, but the kind that makes my muscles ache and then grow stronger.

The prose is musical, it ebbs and flows. It reminds me of Beethoven's Fifth Symphony that within seconds lifts your soul, except the joy in the pages of this story lasts longer.

I have reached the emotional scene of the evening that Annette and her son, after years of misunderstanding, find their way into each other's hearts. Annette loved nothing in life more than this rebellious boy, who just like her seeks freedom and perfection. They sit hour after hour, far into the night, speaking to one another:

> And they continued to do so later, from one room to the other, when at last they decided to go to bed. Then, in the middle of the night, he got up and went in his bare feet into Annette's room. He sat down in a low chair by her bedside. They did not talk anymore. They only needed to be near each other.

My eyes well up as I feel the tenderness between the two. How can someone make up such powerful scenes? How can a writer chisel such strong emotions? He lifts me and drops me in a different place and time where I see sincerity, courage and love.

I write in my journal—the one I call the White Notebook because it has a leather white jacket—that I want to write too, even though it won't be as powerful as Rolland. But I want to write because other writings nurtured my imagination, gave me wings to fly and expanded my world.

And then, I feel the urge to speak to Katy, my friend who has already finished the book. Katy and I don't have the vocabulary yet to discuss how the book is molding us but we wonder what kind of a mind would give birth to such magical characters.

#

Katy and I pick up the conversation decades later after a shocking discovery when we look up our beloved author on the internet. What pops up leaves us speechless: a picture of Rolland with Joseph Stalin.

The black-and-white photo, taken on June 28, 1935, shows the two men sitting at a table against a wood-paneled wall. Stalin, in a bright buttoned-up shirt, looks straight into the camera. Rolland is slightly slouched, his bony hands are on top of one another. He looks into the distance.

We learn that he wrote Stalin letters calling him "Dear Comrade Stalin." Was he just a leftist intellectual thinking Stalin could save France from Nazi Germany, or did he remain a devoted sympathizer of a mass murderer?

Katy and I were victims of an ideology very similar to communism that perished the lives of our loved ones and crushed our spirits. In total confusion, I search for an explanation. I come across a review that answers a different question. A Goodreads review in Persian—in fact, the only review of *The Enchanted Soul*—perhaps by a woman my age, finally articulates what I was unable to grasp at such young age: that Annette was the identity that my generation needed as a woman and a mother during a time that we were ripped off of our own identity by a war, a revolution and zealotry.

I search for more. Even other reviews in English are written by Iranian women. A woman named Shadi, whose name means happiness in Persian, writes that Annette "is not an ordinary nurturing woman, but more an arrow of wisdom for the ones who are seeking it."

But how do I separate the writer from the writing? I learn the creator of such indelible characters was married to a Russian woman, Lenin invited him to Russia and he interviewed Stalin. He was also friends with Gandhi and Sigmund Freud and corresponded with both men. He was known as a humanist.

I decide that I may never know why Rolland sympathized with an autocrat. But I know that his writing moved me in such a profound way that nearly four decades later I can close my eyes and reach out for Annette with a knot in my throat.

#

It's Friday. I go back to Shamsi's apartment, where every single wall is covered with bookshelves, to pick my next summer read. Her husband, a medical doctor by training, collected works of fiction. Shamsi saw him today. "Maybe they'll release him," she tells me. The grooves on her face tell me the toll his incarceration has taken on her.

The framed portraits of her three adult children beam on the table with white smiles. I pass the shelf packed with Persian poetry books that are part of every household. I sift through the novels, looking for a read that would suck me in the same way *The Enchanted Soul* did and spit me out a different person. I settle on *Jean Christophe*, the book that earned Rolland's 1915 Nobel Peace Prize in Literature.

Peg Boyers

Poet, Editor

Driven

My first poems were written in the car on a primitive laptop in 1995, the year our youngest son began boarding school. I was driven to write (literally and figuratively) on weekend journeys to New Hampshire where my husband and I would stay in a hotel and spend some time with our son, occasionally alone, frequently with his friends, at meals or school activities. It was our first autumn as premature empty-nesters, speeding off to visit him every weekend a matter of survival—ours, not his.

Our son's leaving home at fifteen was a change in our lives of seismic proportions—I felt its sweeping effects profoundly in body and mind. For many years I had worked as Executive Editor of Salmagundi Magazine, reading and commenting on poems, never aspiring to be a poet myself. But following my son's departure, when the various continental shifts in my physical and emotional make-up settled, poems—or rather "poems"—started to manifest themselves as phrases and images occupying my brain, demanding my attention. I began taking them down diligently, as if by dictation. They were not poems yet, but rather stanzas and passages, and they were not focused on the experience of having our son living away from home. They were not poems of loss or grief or of what I suppose some women feel when their children leave home—relief or liberation. They were about my own childhood, a subject which, as I learned from the painfully bad poems that came out, I was ill-equipped to address. Nevertheless, I persisted—writing lines, making lists of impressions and pressing memories I needed somehow to tame, if not resolve. To my astonishment I found that my recurring concerns were the familiar themes of Literature: Family/Identity/Marriage/Motherhood. But the poems in which I attempted to make something of these themes were weighed down by what seemed the embarrassing banality of my life. I felt unable to discover in that banality something genuine, worthy of the poems I might hope to write.

DOI: 10.4324/9781003516118-19

I needed to find a way to translate that material, or rather translate what was essential in it, into something like poetry, about which I thought I knew a great deal, but about which, as a writer, I was fairly clueless. Born in Venezuela to a Cuban mother and Irish father, spending my childhood in Cuba, Indonesia, Nigeria, Libya and Italy, I have always been accustomed to thinking and expressing myself in more than one language. Among those languages, the ones spoken in the countries where I resided the longest have remained dominant—Spanish, Italian and English—and they are the languages shared by the members of my family, all of us employing all three naturally when with and apart from one another, slipping in and out of them interchangeably and as a matter of course.

For all of us, growing up as we did, translation was more than a necessity. It was our way of reinforcing our membership in a peculiar clan. Say "you must be joking" in English and it means one thing, say it in Italian and it means another; say it in Spanish with a Cuban inflection and it will sound at once more playful and more severe. Drawing upon all of these meanings, using them all at once, was a family habit practiced with ease, even by the youngest among us. Our family humor had much to do with multi-lingual wordplay and silliness, our family in-jokes mostly consisting of misappropriations and deliberate, mischievous subversions of ordinary usage. There were no writer-models in my extended family, none in either set of ancestors, but we were all translators, spontaneously translating and transposing our family lore, the tri-lingual jokes and sayings a tribal code and source of fun. Birthday poems, anniversary doggerel and rollicking epithalamia would reliably issue from this shared sense that writing and translation were for pleasure.

#

My own time in boarding school was very different from our son's. I was far from my family, enrolled in a school on the outskirts of Rome, and had ample time to explore the city and to further immerse myself in all things Italian. By the time our son went away to boarding school, decades after my own adolescence, I had been reading Natalia Ginzburg's work in Italian for many years, and I knew the neighborhood of Piazza Navona where she lived very well. Twice I interviewed her at her Rome apartment in 1990, shortly before she died, and even translated a few of her essays and plays into English. Often I thought about her and her life. Often I thought that though we were very different, there was a sense in which we were sisters, and when she cooked me lunch one day, and spoke to me about intimate matters as if we were already close, I felt an affinity with her that I have rarely felt with any other writer.

Though it may seem improbable, when I came back to my poetry and struggled to make it an expression of what was deepest and truest in me, I began to experiment with Ginzburg as my muse and as my subject matter. Using her life and work as a vessel into which I could pour my own awakening emotions and urgent needs for expression came to me as a natural solution. Why not draw upon her relationship to her father and siblings to explore the troubling thoughts I was having about the effects of disobedience and the necessity of lies in my own family? Why not explore my own crisis of faith through what I imagined might have been—had to be—hers? Why not explore the terrors I felt throughout my pregnancy by imagining Ginzburg's relationship with her own disabled daughter, to whom she had introduced me at her Rome apartment?

And so it was that I put aside my early poems about my family and apprenticed myself to Ginzburg, or rather to her work, as she was no longer alive when I wrote my poems about her. She had written novels, stories, essays and plays but only one poem during her lifetime. My new vocation, I realized, was to write *her* poems about *her* family and *her* experience, to write poems *for* her. It was in *her* life and its circumstances—her Italian spaces, her Italian light—that I found the inspiration to develop a voice of my own.

Once that inspiration took hold there was no stopping me. Every Friday afternoon as we drove across Vermont to New Hampshire to see our son, I would bang away at my laptop all the way, and then turn around on Sunday afternoon and write for four more hours all the way home. Something about being enclosed in a private place, barely aware of the continuously changing landscape outside the window, something about those luxurious four-hour blocks of undisturbed writing time, made it the ideal space for my imaginary excursion through another person's life, allowing me to write some thirty poems over the course of two years. It's as if the clarity and stability of the process taking place in my mind and on the page were made possible by the blur passing me by outside the speeding vehicle. I don't think what was going on outside was irrelevant at all; rather, it provided a usefully inert surround in which my poems could breathe and grow unencumbered.

Though I was turning out what seemed to me promising poems— innocently, elatedly—I knew that I needed instruction. My good fortune was that a writer I greatly admired was teaching a poetry workshop at the New York State Summer Writers Institute at Skidmore College, and that he welcomed me into his class. The first of my poems that he saw in the workshop had nothing to do with Ginzburg and was relegated, upon the instructor's recommendation, to the "circular file." My second one was better, but nothing special. More or less at once I saw that I needed Ginzburg's sane lucidity, her sharp, austere, sometimes caustic Italian to help me find my own voice in English, and by week two of the workshop

I was writing Ginzburg poems, solidly in her life in the Italian Abruzzi region, writing the letters I imagined she would have sent to her husband Leone, a member of the anti-fascist resistance who was tortured and died in prison.

Soon after, I began to work with the poet Frank Bidart at the same Summer Writers Institute. As a writer of dramatic monologues he seemed to me an ideal person with whom to study as I continued to work my way through a long sequence of poems in the voice of another writer. As I followed Natalia through two wars, two marriages, a career as writer and editor, her eventual illness and death, I tried in each poem to employ a new form to match the subject I hoped to explore. This series of poems, begun in 1997 in response to prompts from my Writers Institute teachers, came together in 2002 as my first book, *Hard Bread*. In writing that book, I learned that as a poet what I most wished to do was to throw my voice, to enter into the perspective of other human beings, to adopt and make credible a persona and to allow that persona to speak almost as if I were speaking for myself. Almost.

#

After I wrote my Ginzburg poems for *Hard Bread*, writing poems became much more difficult, in that I knew it was time to turn to my own life and my own issues without the grid of Ginzburg's life as an overlay for my own. By inhabiting her life and circumstances I had been able to say very intimate things about myself and my own family, things I had been unable to access, let alone openly articulate. The grid was, obviously, a veil, and behind that veil I could, without embarrassment, cry, laugh, grimace or stick my tongue out, self-mockingly. I still miss that grid, that concealing veil.

It's been over twenty years now since the publication of *Hard Bread*. In the meantime, I have had ample time to face my earliest "poems." Some I have managed to bring to life; others have died a quiet death in the process and the world is no sadder for the loss of them. I've since moved on to other projects, getting my inspiration from a variety of sources, driven in a different sense to get to the bottom of this or that issue that presents itself. Some poems are obviously autobiographical in origin; others take their cues from works of art which, seen and cherished as they have been in the museums I have visited and revisited throughout my life, are also intrinsic components of my autobiography.

My most recent book, *The Album*, takes its title from the painter, Edouard Vuillard, and is an entire collection of ekphrastic poems, inspired by, responding to paintings by nineteen artists, from Max Beckmann to Lucian Freud and Albrecht Durer. Though *Honey With*

Tobacco, my second book, is rooted in my Venezuelan and Cuban past, it strays into other domains, and contains a sequence in which intimate questions of my own life as a mother are viewed through the lens of Christian iconography. My third book, *To Forget Venice,* goes back to a period when I landed in Venice at age thirteen and stayed there with my family for nearly two years. But though I began to write that book with purely autobiographical intentions, it follows the trajectory of a person ever fascinated by and drawn back to "La Serenissima" over many years and engages with others who have done the same—so that there are poems spoken in the voices of John Ruskin, Mrs. Casanova and Titian's Magdalena, among others. Though Natalia is no longer my main source of inspiration, there is always another grid somewhere to lay over my own experience, another veil or mask to grab from the shadows and don.

It's fair to say that all my poems are persona poems and that often the voice of the poem's speaker resembles very much that of one Peg Boyers. Other times the imagined speaker is another writer or artist or historical personage, or perhaps a figure in a painting begging to be translated into another medium. When romping in the elysian fields of the imagination it's impossible to overstate the freedom one has to draw either faithfully from life or to make up—or steal—what one needs to fill in the picture one has set out to paint. It's a liberating enterprise when it's going well, even if the task at hand is hard to accomplish. Of course, no one is driving me to do this peculiar thing; no one needs me to do it. And yet, the compulsion is there, and it seems to me to have something at least to do with the fascination with language and languages, the need to translate one thing into another, to consider always what is lost and what is gained in the transaction.

The son we drove to see every weekend at boarding school the year I was driven to begin writing poetry is now forty-five, and his splendid, sometimes turbulent, movement through adolescence and early manhood has continued to provide rich inspiration for me in life and in poetry. By what light and space do I work now? My study until recently has been shaded by an enormous mulberry tree so thick with branches that even in winter when it lost its leaves, its shade barely subsided. This Fall the branches weighed so hard on my study's roof that the corner eaves snapped off. Our kindly neighbor had the tree cut down and now a brilliant, Eastern light glares through my mornings. I am not accustomed to such illumination. My current challenge is to learn to navigate this bright terrain, scan it for useful rays. Maybe nab one—or two—and translate them onto the page.

Sigrid Nunez

Novelist

Preface to an Autobiography

I like the way Rousseau declares in the first sentence of his autobiography that he is about to do something that has never been done before and that will never be done again.

The problem with any first sentence, said Joan Didion, is that you're stuck with it. Everything else is going to flow out of that sentence. And by the time you've laid down the first *two* sentences, your options are all gone.

Before beginning, too many options. Then, in the next breath, none.

When you can't sleep, goes an old cure for insomnia, start telling yourself the story of your life. For some reason, writer's block has always felt to me like a kind of insomnia.

I like that Norman Mailer said there's a touch of writer's block in a writer's work every day.

I don't remember who said, Insomnia is the inability to forget.

When you're having trouble writing, get up, go out, take a walk in the street. You will discover that certain streets exist precisely for this purpose. Once, I saw a man—homeless by the look of him—digging through the trash. He pulled out a couple of sheets of newspaper, examined them, and threw them back. Fishing deeper, he hauled up a magazine, squinted at the cover, and threw it back. Shit, he said, walking away. There ain't nothing to read in these fucking cans anymore.

Rousseau goes on to say that he has embellished the story of his life only to fill a void when his memory failed. But of course he never gives you the heads-up.

Never write "I don't remember," Editor says; it undermines your authority.

But write as if you remember everything and Reader will smell a rat.

I like the student in my graduate fiction-writing class who said, I've read your novels and there's one thing I have to ask: Do you make some of that stuff up?

DOI: 10.4324/9781003516118-20

I like that Allen Ginsburg told a teenager who wanted to know what he should write about that he should write about his love for his friends.

I once made the mistake of writing about a love too soon after it was over. Forgetting Chekhov's advice that you should sit down to write only when you feel as cold as ice.

How can a man who knows nothing about love be a great novelist? a character in a novel by J. M. Coetzee says about a character named John Coetzee.

I like that Virginia Woolf said, Everything I read these days, including my own work, seems to me too long.

That Borges said, Unlike the novel, a short story may be, for all purposes, essential.

But not that Jeanette Winterson said, I think long books are rude.

Not that Céline said, Novels are something like lace, an art that went out with the convent.

More and more, I like the idea of a pen name.

Sugared Nouns was the computer's suggestion, after spell-checking my name.

Some writers use pen names so that they can be more truthful; others, so that they can tell more lies.

I like how Lily Tomlin used to introduce one part of her act: The following skit is about my parents. I have changed their names to protect their identities.

You can start with fiction or start with documentary, according to Jean-Luc Godard. Either way, you will inevitably find the other.

I like the sliver of ice in the heart that Graham Greene thought every writer must have. I have it.

And the grain of stupidity Flannery O'Connor said the writer of fiction can't do without. I have that, too.

I like that Alan Bennett said, For a writer, nothing is ever quite as bad as it is for other people, because, however dreadful, it may be of use.

Oncologist says, That doesn't sound like any writer *I* know.

I like John Banville's paraphrase of Bennett: Writers don't suffer as much as other people.

An enormous stroke of luck is how García Márquez described his cancer diagnosis, for it goaded him to start writing his autobiography.

There is always a sheet of paper. There is always a pen. There is always a way out, wrote H. L. Mencken. Who nevertheless hoped that his life would not last too long.

Write . . . paper . . . pencil are said to have been the dying words of the poet Heine. Unless they were: Of course God will forgive me; that's his job, as has also been reported.

I like that, at the end of his life, Darwin said he wished that he had read more poetry.

That Keynes said he wished that he had drunk more champagne.

That Chekhov said, It's a long time since I drank champagne, then drained his glass and died.

I like last words. Beethoven: I shall hear in Heaven.

Käthe Kollwitz: Good luck, everyone.

Bring me a ladder. Quickly, a ladder! (Gogol)

And nutty epitaphs: I know not everyone is unhappy about this.

I wanted to write a comic novel, then realized I had my own life to hand.

Sugared Nouns: My Life and Death as a Writer.

Once you start on the road to autobiography, fretted Calvino, where do you stop?

I can tell the story of my life in just four words. Good times, bad times.

There will always be lacemakers. There will always be convents.

But about you, my love, I will never feel as cold as ice.

Permissions Line: TK [Permissions request and email thread with Joy Harris Agency and Penguin Random House have been submitted with MS materials]

Marilyn Martin

Psychiatrist, Psychoanalyst, Daughter

Writing and Rescue

On May 21, 1962, my thirteen-year-old brother, David, collapsed from an asthma attack. My father tried to revive him but was unsuccessful, and David died. I was five.

My parents, who had five other young children to raise, were overwhelmed with the kind of grief that only parents who have lost a child know.

The grief seeped into every aspect of our lives. My mother became depressed and wore black until she reunited with David in death, decades later. My father, who also had asthma, was guilt-ridden and had bouts of anger to manage the grief. Every Sunday, after church, we visited David's grave, always taking the same route the hearse took on his burial day. The grief pounded us siblings, committed that we were to be good children and not stress our parents further. They had enough to bear, suffering headaches and other symptoms of unresolved grief. I accompanied my mother to the emergency room with hypertension crises. The hours waiting in the emergency room bred fantasies in which I saw and healed patients quickly.

Being raised by a depressed mother has been shown to affect children. Some become depressed, others have attachment issues. Many others develop rescue fantasies, like my own in the emergency room. My drive to write—the effort to solve the pain of depressed parents—feels like a compulsion rather than a conscious choice.

My first book, *Saving Our Last Nerve: The Black Woman's Path to Mental Health,* was written as a promise I made to my mother. When she was slipping away from dementia, I shared with her how devastating it was to lose her. I promised my mother I would write a book to help guide others through their grief. If I, a psychiatrist and budding psychoanalyst, was having such difficulty letting go, imagine others' journeys.

My second book, in process, is on parental grief. Interviewing parents who are grieving puts me in direct interaction with the people I am

DOI: 10.4324/9781003516118-21

trying so earnestly to rescue. I am repeating with them, over and over, what was so painful in my life: the loss of my mother through our family's unresolved grief and depression. My perpetual wish is that grief and depression might be resolved and I can have my healthy mother back. I repeat this wish, while seeking to save as many parents as I can, always hoping that this time it will be different.

I write because there is a whole community of grieving and depressed parents to save and maybe, just maybe, I will heal my own wounds in the process.

Jean McGarry

Writer, Professor

On Writer's Block: A Meditation on Sadism

In a writing life extending to nearly half a century, I have never experienced writer's block in its classic form: writer sits down in front of a blank page, and the page stays blank. But, over the course of writing and publishing ten books of fiction, I've encountered something quite odd: a mysterious but predictable arrest, not *before* writing, but after seeing what I *had* written. It was in the course of a long analysis that I came to identify its cause, and also realized how powerful this arrest could be.

Early in my writing life, a teacher—the late novelist John Hawkes— had pinpointed the source of most imaginative writing. The fiction-writer, he said, was taking—and had to take—"revenge for the indignities of childhood."

I took this in, but somehow the force of it eluded me, even as I enacted my own revenge in my first book, *Airs of Providence,* a story collection steeped in my childhood memories. I was somehow able to write this book without equating its composition with an act of violence against the McGarrys of Providence.

The book was published three decades ago by a university press with a small circulation, so I didn't imagine my parents would ever find it, nor had I ever seen them as my readers. But an odd splash in the Rhode Island paper of record brought it to their attention, and their (and the neighbors') reading of *Airs* caused quite a commotion. It was only in their hurt and outrage that I saw how what seemed funny to me felt like a knife in the back to them. Reviewers and other neutral readers confirmed that this book was indeed a targeted missile, a tale of the daily life of a miserable, fractious, chaotic family, recorded by an oddly oblivious child. My parents were hurt, and they were angry, and they had their own way of getting even.

My father told me that people in *his* family knew how to *keep* a secret. (A poet confided to me that, upon offering his childhood memoir

DOI: 10.4324/9781003516118-22

to his dying father, the latter told the poet that he would have had him "knee-capped," if the manuscript weren't so poorly written that it'd never see the light of day.) Eventually, my parents got over this first round, and hardened themselves to—and even collaborated with—my writing that followed, where my pen always seemed to land in the old neighborhood, "telling tales."

So far, so good, but in these later books, things went downhill, and it took me a long time to see what was at the root of an ever-returning writing battle.

If Hawkes was right, and what drives a writer is revenge, then that same impulse could equally well shut the work down. It's not so easy to avenge the indignities of childhood and get away with it. It's not even a simple matter to dredge up those indignities. Mining painful scenes from childhood is painful; mining them with the aim of getting even seems a recipe for inhibition or prohibition.

As I've noted, my experience with writer's block is less of a drastic work stoppage than a sudden and painful nausea or revulsion, which halts composition for at least a day. It comes at the sight—in revision—of a lapse in the writing: a vague, dull, or misplaced word. How, if I call myself a writer, could I be this stupid? This happens most often in writing novels. I've written six. I start out easily, working freely, composing scenes and chapters with a sense of who my people are and where they're heading. I can get the full draft down in that first flush, whether it's ten, fifteen or twenty chapters. It might take months to get from page one to the end, but the handwritten draft is not subject to enactments of revolt and self-censorship. Rather, *this* destructive work begins the moment I try to convert the hand-written pages to a typescript. Even then, I can transfer what I've written, compressing it a bit, as I go along.

The trouble really starts a bit later, when—pen in hand—I take up the typescript and begin reading it, word by word, page by page, thinking about the prospect of a book. Things go rapidly downhill from here, as revision follows slashing revision. Stylistically, my typical early draft, written in a free, loose and full style will be gutted so roughly that something that started out with flesh ends up bone dry. Many times, in the course of *seeing what I've done,* I've lost heart entirely and been unable to go on.

I remember once taking the typescript of my second book, *The Very Rich Hours,* on a cross-country train trip, thinking I'd found the ideal time to plunge into the manuscript, undisturbed, and draw out its essence. The train hadn't reached Philadelphia's 30th Street Station before I was in despair at the mess I'd made. I decided, an hour and a half into a three-day journey, to trash the book.

This sequence—serene first draft, tortured revision—has dogged my every novel. Toward the end of the process, I usually recognize that

I have turned the narrative into a digest, something so compact that the surface cracks with tension, and has also acquired an admonitory tone, as if the sentences were all imperatives. Oddly, this work stoppage and contraction rarely happens with short stories, which come out, the first time, almost the way they'll look in print. For this writer, if a story starts with the right sentence—voice and rhythm—the story will be finished when the last word is written. Novels are different, and why could that be?

I have mostly been a writer of stories, perhaps for many reasons, and my stories have gradually grown in scope to cover something of a novel's time. They are condensed, compressed, and move fast. They're done before I half realize what I've written, or what it might mean. This act of sprinting, racing start to finish, is a natural mode. The story might take a couple of weeks of ingathering, but it's a steady process of laying sentence upon sentence. By contrast, a novel is broody, slow, accumulative. It's hard to write one without knowing what you're doing, without seeing what it is you're really writing about.

As a writer who started out vengeful, but really didn't want to be seen—or see herself—as a critic, I had a problem. I learned in my own psychoanalysis that my extreme reaction to less-than-perfect diction was probably a reaction to something hidden, a recognition that I was doing something bad. What struck me as inept, or bland, or wordy—a stylistic flaw—was also, or even mainly, a sign that I was enacting revenge. I knew there had to be something else going on besides an act of stylistic brightening, when there were occasions when I could look at the same reviled page with pleasure, perhaps replacing a word or two. The proof of the pudding came when, after multiple, painful revisions, I would notice—if I had the nerve to look back—that the first "bad" draft wasn't all that different from the last, perfect one. That should have told me something: that the self-judgment was censorship. But I didn't analyze the problem until I was in analysis, and the matter came up again and again, whenever I was at work on a novel.

And the process, to this day, is always the same, always grueling; grueling because I'm torn between the need to write this particular book and the almost equally strong need not to. The punishment I can call down upon myself for the wrong word, or a scene not fully fleshed out in the first pass, is extreme. But I always go back—or almost always. The struggle is intense and exhausting. The desire to write must be slightly stronger than the desire to stifle.

It's interesting to me that the problem occurs on the surface level— the word level, the same level that analysts use to uncover defenses, drive derivatives, traces of repression. Using breaks in the surface of words to approach the concealed depth. Analysts stick to the patient's words, looking for moments when the flow is interrupted, or stopped and suddenly re-started somewhere else: a jump, a reversal, a transition, something that shows a pattern not obvious to the patient—a pattern emerging from a deeper level, a conflict, usually, or a defense against an unwanted thought or feeling. The analyst's way of working is so close to my experience of writer's block that it still amazes me. I am both analyst and analysand in writing and reading my work. Sometimes I don't like what I see, but I don't know why. As a writer, I use my stylistic training to avoid and suppress; as a student of a psychoanalysis, and as an analysand, I try to understand the struggle, and why it's timed for the final stages of bringing a book into the world.

I have a story called "A Full House" in a collection entitled *Ocean State* where a woman, returning home at the news of her father's suicide, finds that he's left her five letters, each hidden in different spot in their family home, where he has been living alone. One by one, the daughter finds the letters as she muses on what she'll say in her eulogy about her famous father. The daughter reviews a lifetime of scenes where she's been shamed, humiliated, antagonized and turned, sometimes, into a substitute wife by this arrogant man, who is, by the way, a psychiatrist. She sees how her own adult life has been overshadowed and oppressed by this parent.

This was a hard story for me to write. I loathed the cold, brutal tone I'd chosen for the narration; I wrote and rewrote the contents of the father's five letters. I couldn't get those letters right, and the sight of the early drafts appalled me—they seemed so naked, a plea for pity. I also couldn't really focus on the character of the daughter. Was she just a doormat? Did she ever fight back? What was she going to say about him, now that she had the chance?

Looking back, this seems a case where the material itself—the situation and the characters—were upsetting to the writer: my character was aflame with rage, but was this rage ever going to erupt? Did the writer have the nerve to let it? But it was primarily the words that struck like poisoned darts, causing me to stop, to dig them out, to replace them, to start over. I made many, many drafts, and the story took over half a year to write. It still has an ambiguous ending.

The last scene has the daughter, Patricia Pierce, waiting in a cathedral for her father's memorial service to start; and then, when it does start, she unseals and reads the five letters. The church is full of bigshots, because the doctor-father was a local celebrity. As Patricia reads the letters, we hear what they say—either their exact words, or a summary—then, she rises to go to the pulpit. We don't hear *her* words, her eulogy—and perhaps that was a dodge—but we do know how she feels, and that something in her life is now very different.

An earlier version of the story includes a letter full of the father's scorn for domestic life, and his condescension toward his wife and daughters. Through his bluff manner, we can see the pain he's in. Before Patricia reads this letter, and while people are marching up to receive communion—in this early draft—she even feels the physical presence of her father, hovering:

> During this bustle, Patricia felt the touch of an arm on her back and at her shoulder, but no bodily warmth. First, tentative and weightless, then she felt the contraction, almost painful in its intensity. She opened her summer purse and took out the letters.

In the final version of the story, after I cut all the hateful and pathetic letters, there's nothing personal at all in the doctor's first four letters—although they're mocking and contemptuous—but the fifth letter shows him playing his last card, a trick card. It's a test for Patricia, but also a desperate stay against what he knows to be true: that simply by outliving him, Patricia will have the last word.

The story, in its printed version, is as fierce as I could make it. But the sight of it—of what I was saying—was so upsetting to me that I revised and revised, erasing and erasing, subtracting and adding, doing and undoing. It's a miracle I ever finished it. I dedicated the book to my analyst because, without her, a few things in this book, including this story, would never have come to light.

Nancy J. Chodorow

Theorist, Teacher, Clinician

To Tell People What I Think

As a reader, in psychoanalysis and in the social sciences, I love narratives: clinical cases, interview studies, ethnographies. But as a writer, I'm a theorist. I find linkages among ideas and observed phenomena in the everyday sociocultural and psychological world.

My writing career did not begin auspiciously. My father was a physicist, and my mind works like his. He once told me that while he was not a theorist (in physics, the theory stakes are high!), he could hear lectures in different theoretical arenas months or years apart and then could imagine an "instrument" that combined them. Like my father, I find networks and connections among diverse ideas and phenomena. Fascinated by theory, and telling people what I think.

But growing up, I didn't know that writing could be a way to tell people what I think. This did not seem to be what "writing" meant. As a young child, I took words, rhyme, rhythm and music for granted. I was read children's stories and knew nursery rhymes, A.A. Milne's poetry volumes and lots of songs. Then came my voracious reading of children's fiction, chapter books that I was given as presents or borrowed from the library. When I got older, I was sometimes asked to write in social studies. But that wasn't called writing; it was a "paper." "Writing" was what happened in English classes, and it was a challenge.

Here, my prehistory may have been a burden. While my father was a physicist, my parents' world included, in addition to scientists, well-known social scientists, historians, poets, novelists and cultural commentators. When told to "write a poem" in high school English, I froze. My mother consulted close friends, a well-known novelist and a poetry professor, to find a graduate student tutor for me. When I thought I might study history, my model was my father's best friend since college, by then a leading American historian.

Sitting for placement in honors English, I was told: "Write about irony." What's irony?

DOI: 10.4324/9781003516118-23

In (non-honors) English: "Write a joke." The psychopathology of everyday life was to be experienced, not written about!

Yet as a college sophomore I persisted, pursuing a major in "History and Literature." Upon reading my first essay, my tutor did not believe I had even read *Le Neveu de Rameau*, and I received a C+ in my nineteenth-century novel course: "Write about character in . . ." Character?

Then I found the social sciences! My grades and enthusiasm soared. In a course nicknamed "Stones and Bones" (archaeology and physical anthropology), I got an A+. Writing was no longer a seemingly unattainable craft in which you could only reflect on character, or notice style and rhythm. You could write about something in the world. I switched majors.

I started to like writing, then, when I was writing about something that really mattered to me, though it took a while for me to know what the *about* was; to feel it, know its force and name it. Retrospectively, I can put together the pieces, remembering the books that affected me: Freud's *Civilization and Its Discontents*, read in freshman history, and, the following summer, discovering on my parents' bookshelves Erik Erikson's *Childhood and Society* and Oscar Lewis' psychological ethnography, *The Children of Sanchez*. I recognized myself and my history in Erikson's Sam, a Jewish boy from New York who notices the cultural expectations of the gentile San Francisco Bay area. Before we moved West when I was three, I had asked my mother, "Will we only have *friends*, and no *family*, in California?" I was finding my voice, my words and, not negligibly, my passions. My subject became psyche, culture and society; the theoretical underpinnings of each, and the connections among them. I had ideas, and I wanted readers to know what I think.

I still want readers to know what I think, but the greater truth is that I want them to know what is *right*. Implicitly, as I see it, I've always written for two audiences: on the one side, sociologists, anthropologists and feminists who need to recognize what comes emotionally from within. They make a big mistake if they think that lives are primarily socially, politically or culturally determined. On the other side, psychoanalysts need to know that psychic life draws from and is shaped by the socio-political-cultural-gendered-racial-ethnic.

I first applied this perspective to feminism. My dissertation (which, with very little revision, became my first book, *The Reproduction of Mothering*) began with straightforward questions. Why is there an extensive literature on mothers and sons, and *nothing* on mothers and daughters? Why are *mothers* blamed for what's wrong with their sons? For what's wrong in the *world*? Look at the language taken for granted: "a generation of vipers," "maternal deprivation," "maternal overprotection," "schizophrenogenic mothers."

Psychological anthropology and psychoanalytic sociology did not provide an answer, so I turned to psychoanalysis itself. But there, also, no one had thought to wonder: how *do* women become mothers? *The Reproduction of Mothering* is what I discovered, though not what I set out to find. The book opens with a two-word sentence, "Women mother." And it goes on to puzzle this:

> Because of the seemingly natural connection between women's child-bearing and lactation capacities and their responsibility for childcare, and because humans need extended care in childhood, women's mothering has been taken for granted . . . by social scientists, by many feminists, and certainly by those opposed to feminism. As a result . . . it is rarely analyzed. This book analyzes women's mothering.

And *The Reproduction of Mothering* closes, "Women mother daughters who, when they become women, mother."

There is a risk when you write in order to tell people what is important for them to know, especially when they don't want to hear it. I had difficulty getting a first academic position, and *The Reproduction of Mothering*, now seen as foundational, was rejected by one press whose reviewer commented forcefully that psychoanalysis has no evidential or research basis. Even the book's eventual publisher wondered, "Is 'mothering' a word?"

Yes, mothering is a word, and more. It's an activity, an identity, a relationship, a process, as is writing. For me, writing is an activity and identity through which I seek to achieve precise meaning, and to convey something that I care about to others. I want to write with the greatest clarity of meaning I can muster, to convey what I think and feel about something in the world. That is the understanding of writing that saved, or created, me as a writer.

For me, writing is not an art, not a craft; I do not consciously pay attention to sounds or the crafting of sentences. Yet, I have long known that I subvocalize as I read, and in writing this essay, I realized that I also do so when I write. I am musical and a late-life choral singer; the sounds and rhythms of words and phrases must be somewhere in there. Perhaps even when I tell the world that they need to know about the unconscious mother-daughter relationship and its role in maternal identity.

In graduate school I studied ethnomethodology. Its subject is what is taken for granted in everyday life, just as psychoanalysis begins from the premise that we cannot take our conscious thoughts for granted, and anthropology from the premise that we cannot take our own culture for granted. These fields all meet me where I live: entwined with telling people what they may not want to know is the notice I give to what's taken for granted. I have told sociologists that people's lives are shaped not only by society and culture, but created through personal meaning. I've told psychoanalysts to pay attention not just to homosexuality and so-called "perversions" but to pay attention to heterosexuality, too.

I am a contrarian, but aim to be one who builds bridges, between psychoanalysis and the social sciences and between competing psycho-analytic traditions. In psychoanalysis, in social science, in feminism, and in writing, I share what I want readers to notice. I share what I think.

Thomas H. Ogden

Teacher, Writer, Psychoanalyst

Why I Write

Both the art of being an analyst and the art of being a father are, for me, inseparable from the art of writing. To put this the other way around, learning how to write is an integral part of how I go about trying to become a better father than my father was for me, and a better analyst than my analysts were for me. I take the three—becoming a better writer, a better father and a better analyst—as interwoven responsibilities. My father's having been a better father to me than his father was to him, and my becoming a better father than he was, seem to me to be essential parts of the way human progress is made.

I write analytic essays, literary essays and fiction because writing in these genres teaches me what I think and gives me a sense of who I am. I do not know what I am going to write when I sit down to write; I find out what I think in the process of writing it. Thinking in the process of writing is a principal medium in which I become more the person, the father, the analyst I would like to be: a person who aspires to (and inspires) imaginative thinking, artistic expression, critical judgment, truthfulness, and tact.

For me, the art of being an analyst involves the art of writing—the two are inseparable, each opens the door to the other. Writing is like dreaming in that it is a medium in which I think and talk to myself in ways that I cannot do in any other form. Also, like dreaming, it keeps me alive in my work as a psychoanalyst, for I find that I have to be creating something of my own (to come more fully into being myself) as I am immersed in trying to help a patient engage in creating something unique of his or her own (in coming more fully into being).

Part of the difficulty in writing well lies in the fact that writing of any sort—analytic essay, literary essay, poetry, fiction—is autobiographical. After all, where do feelings, thoughts and responses originate other than from oneself, one's past experiences, including one's fantasies? Consequently, when I write I put my private world on the page. The more I am

DOI: 10.4324/9781003516118-24

able to do so, the more I am able to bring a situation to life in the writing. But "opening myself up" in the act of writing is not enough. I must do something original with my writing. I must find a way of capturing a situation in my own way, a way that bears my own mark, which I create in the way I use language. And that mark is a living thing that is alive only when I am writing. When I'm not writing, I am someone preparing to write again.

The analysand and I undergo different sorts of experiencing as we are engaged in the art of psychoanalysis: our roles are different and the sorts of artfulness entailed in those roles differ. Writing, as a part of the art of psychoanalysis, does not explain why anyone does anything or feels anything; it describes, and does so in a very particular way. Experience does not come in words; it is utterly inarticulate, so one cannot write the experience one has had in an analytic session. Writing must create something of its own that reflects what happens in a session. (A transcript of an analytic session utterly fails to convey what it was like to be there in the session.) So, as an analytic writer, I face the task and the opportunity to engage in the art of writing to create (for myself and the reader) an experience in reading that brings to life something like the experience that occurred in the session. It is extremely difficult to do this well and has required decades to learn how to do it better.

Analytic writing—writing that creates something of its own in the medium of language—is not simply like fiction, it is a form of fiction. The patient who is created in an analytic paper is not the patient who lies down on the analytic writer's couch; the experience with that patient can never be transcribed. The patient in the analytic paper is a character invented by the analytic writer, just as characters are invented by a novelist. Both the characters created by the analytic writer and those created by the novelist are "based on" real people, for it is impossible for writers to create a character that is not derived, at least in part, from their experiences with themselves or with other people. Even the theories developed in analytic writing are fictions. There is no id or ego or superego; there are no beta elements or alpha elements or alpha function; there are no such things as internalization or internal objects; there is no true or false self. Analytic theory is a collection of metaphorical constructs—none of which actually exist. And these metaphors will grow old and tired, and will be replaced by other metaphors.

My principal teachers of writing have not been analytic writers, though I greatly admire Donald Winnicott's writing and consider him to be the finest analytic writer writing in English. My principal teachers have been my university professors of writing composition and the poets, novelists, short story writers and playwrights who have stunned me with what they are able to do with words. I read as a writer. I notice how writers use language: how they create a narrative voice or the voice of a character that I could not have imagined, and to which I could listen forever in rapt attention; how a combination of first-person and third-person narration is made to work when it shouldn't; the turns of phrase and neologisms that are at once natural and staggering. I am humbled by these writers, but I have no wish to imitate them. To try to write the way they do would not only be impossible, it would not be any fun. Writing, though difficult and often trying, is ultimately a pleasurable experience. It is endlessly surprising, puzzling, confounding and fulfilling.

I cannot imagine life without writing. One of the great losses that death will bring is: no more writing. And at the same time, two of the things that make the prospect of death bearable are the joy I take in seeing my son being a better father to his children than I was to him, and my hope that both my sons' experience with me while I found my art as a writer will help them find such a passion for themselves, which they may pass on to their children and students.

Forrest Hamer

Poet, Psychoanalyst

On Bearing and Being Born

February 1966

When my mother was pregnant with the brother
who didn't live,
I wrote a poem that gave me my life.

It could be said that my mother and father gave me my life,
that the families and the times

from which they thrived made me. But in the same way a
child becomes
conscious of the larger world

at six or seven, it was a poem I wrote at nine that made me
conscious
of the inheritance I have been

struggling ever since to realize.

My mother's pregnancy amazed me.

Once, I placed an open ear against her belly and felt
the heat of her
and my brother against it,

her left arm resting above her swollen stomach and the other wrap-
ping my back
as I stood there with my eyes closed.

DOI: 10.4324/9781003516118-25

Because I am deaf in one ear, the sound I strained to know was the music
of some whole world,

the sound I would hear laying my ear against all the other bodies I have loved.
But the poem I wrote was not a poem

of babies, not a poem of hearing private sound, not even a poem about loss,
but a poem about Negroes.

I couldn't make sense of being a Negro, couldn't fully understand
the Negro facts I was memorizing;

the Negro history of the uncountable brought to a developing country
to slave to people who lived now across town; or

the Negro problems still urgent and unsolved. And I don't know how I came
to that problem of history not making sense

by making a poem, a poem not something I had made before, and thought of
only in terms of pleasure.

#

Sometimes at nine there is a new understanding.

#

It wasn't that I didn't understand race. I had known for some time that having dark skin

—even when the dark-skinned were as light as any white—
was grave in this country,

that it marked the boundaries of neighborhoods, churches and schools;
that it was the source of danger

in a world outside of the borders; that it seemed as core to
each other
as each sex or each color of the eyes;

that its power in the country exceeded even God's. But what
I hadn't known
until I was nine, until I became mindful

of the enigmatic problem, was what the matter of dark and light skin
had to do
with my future.

In a world I had newfound abilities to imagine.

#

In one theory of unconsciousness, each child's unconscious is
figured in relation
to the unconscious of the parents,

an enigma which seduces the child into being, even beyond
what parents can conceive.

And each parent's unconscious is figured in turn by the unconscious
of the many
who brought them into being;

so each of us is barely able to know what it is we know, and who.

My mother's pregnancy amazed me

and I think I thought I was making something of my own by making
a life
I had been given

but could not, did not finally want to bear.

#

Sometimes at nine there is a new understanding. In the poem I became

a speaker and
a spoken-to, otherness within me that space where facts and the fantastic

overwhelm
sense. Four three-beat lines in three stanzas, an old song's order
constraining

but consoling,
marching toward the acknowledgment I too was a Negro: I too
understood

something
about the history I was trying to bear, trying to live in spite of, live
with,

live through:
it would not break me, would not beat me down or split me
now in two.

#

There is a brother who didn't live.
There are others, and they are very many.

Now, I hear them.

Carl Phillips

Poet

The Winged Horses Look Like Horses

"it's//a human need, to give to shapelessness/a form."

Why do you write is a question I've been asked many times in my thirty-some years as a publishing poet, and for almost that long I've said I write in order to put a temporary wedge between myself and the unbearable, by which I mean the seemingly unbearable; it's bearable, I'm just not ready—not yet emotionally, psychologically equipped enough—to bear it.

Around the 1980s, when I was writing what would become my first book of poems, the "it" was my being a gay man, a truth which I'd somehow managed to suppress, enough to have ended up married to a woman—a best friend from college whom, yes, I sincerely loved, but had I understood that my attraction to men—in my head, at least—was more than sexual . . . No, had I understood that sexual attraction was hardly to be dismissed as fleeting and ultimately meaningless, i.e., didn't "count," I'd never have gotten married, I'd never have misled anyone, including myself.

My completely amateur sense of how the brain works, when it comes to information, is that it suppresses—stores—information that we're not ready for, what could break us if we reckoned with it too soon; in that sense, suppression is a rescuing force. But it's as if some part of us that I'll *call* the brain also knows that, eventually, we need to face what we've been avoiding, so it begins to deliver that information slant (to borrow from Dickinson)—partly as a release valve for the long-pent-up truth, and partly as an entry point for us to start understanding the truth *as* truth.

The poem tends to know what we don't yet know. Or, more exactly, the subconscious part of us, once it finds its conduit, tends to deliver

DOI: 10.4324/9781003516118-26

what our conscious selves for the moment resist. What, for example, if not my subconscious, led me to choose as epigraph for my first book these lines from *Romans* (8:15), arranged thus:

> for what I would, that do I not;
>   but what I hate, that do I.

—lines that now seem to address very clearly the wrestling between who I wanted to be—who I am—and who I felt I was supposed to be, according to everything I'd read and heard all my life. The book's opening poem, "X," ends with these lines:

> X, not
>
> just for where in my
> life you've landed,
>
> but here too, where
> your ass begins its
>
> half-shy, half-weary
> dividing, where I
>
> sometimes lay my head
> like a flower, and
>
> think I mean something
> by it. X is all I keep
>
> meaning to cross out.

When I look at it now, that final sentence—"X is all I keep meaning to cross out"—clearly speaks to a tug-of-war between an intention to hide/erase something and an ongoing refusal to do so; how could I not see that? What did I *think* I meant, when I wrote those lines? I don't remember. Going back to the opening lines of this essay, I suppose I was trying to give a form to the shapelessness of my identity-in-wobbly-flux . . . That earlier part, though, "where I sometimes lay my head like a flower, and think I mean something by it," speaks of deception—specifically, of being aware of deceiving not only another person but myself as well; I *think* I mean something by it, as opposed to actually meaning it. That part I remember. I can't forget it. I've tried.

What I know for sure is that each time I wrote a poem back then, it felt—to be absolutely frank—the way it felt right after I'd "broken down" and enjoyed the fantasy of sex with another man via the resources available in that pre-internet era: porn magazines, phone chat lines, and in "just" two instances, an actual human being. It felt—right after—as if I'd immediately stepped away from, and could look at, the part of me that had succumbed, that had been weak. I did not recognize the person I saw. Which meant I could walk away and tell myself, "Well, that happened, but not to me, because here I am now, getting on with my day productively." Sex as catharsis, sex also as a catalyst for a dissociation (and a detachment from blame) that, to this day, I believe saved me from suicide—that's how wrenching the turmoil inside me had come to be.

The more wrenching it got, the more poems I wrote. I'd stopped writing, after college; I'd decided it must have been a passing hobby, since I felt no desire to write, and no regrets about that. I see now that I needed the roughly seven years of silence to start processing, if only subconsciously, the various parts of my identity that were just beginning to settle into the configuration of an adult human being fully engaged with his authentic self. It took me a while. As I say, seven years. After which, as if out of nowhere, I began writing poems that bore no resemblance to anything I'd written before, and at a pace I'd never before experienced, as if I'd finally found the language to accommodate what I needed to say and I couldn't say it fast enough or enough times. I wrote a lot of poems for a few years. From here, the correlation is clear between my writing productivity at that time and the steadily decreasing distance between my conscious self—straight, married, voted most popular teacher by my high school students—and my forbidden and "other" queer self.

This is meant as an essay on why I write, not on how I write, but it feels worth mentioning that readers have speculated over the years as to where my sentences, with their tendency toward subordinate clauses, inflected syntax and seemingly ceaseless self-correction/revision come from. There may be truth to the idea that I'm influenced by having studied languages like Greek and Latin, as well as truth to my own assertion that I learned sentence-making from reading earlier prose stylists like Henry James, George Eliot, Marcel Proust, Virginia Woolf . . . but I also think now that I was fashioning for myself a space I could hide inside until I was able to openly be who I needed to be. The sentence, therefore, as camouflage; what else is it, to be camouflaged, if not to be hiding in plain sight for those paying attention? I'd begun paying close attention. Prayer, they say, is a form of attention. So, as I understand it, is psychoanalysis. So too is poetry.

#

So, is this still why I write—to fend off the unbearable?

One of the first fears I had, once I'd come out as gay and I'd settled into what would be a seventeen-year relationship with another man, was: what if I can't write anymore, now that I've answered the elusive riddle of who I am? Of course, my first mistake was thinking that sexual identity was the sum of a self, or that this was the only part of the self to be reckoned with across a lifetime. It's a bit like falling in love and declaring the mystery of love laid to rest forever. And yet, by definition—my own, anyway—abstraction always resists absolute understanding, refuses to be pinned down and disassembled, as opposed, say, to a cake, for which there are recipes, or raising a barn, to which there's a physics and a geometry—we have only to follow the instructions and voilà: a barn, a cake . . .

For better and worse, the governing abstractions of a life (among them love, death, sorrow, freedom, fear, wonder, doubt, rage and joy) turn out to be in constant motion, as is our understanding of them—necessarily, since in a sense we are always becoming different selves and therefore have to revisit and recalibrate our earlier understanding. To stick to love, for example, how I understood it at twelve, say, when my notion of love was confined to what I felt for a pet, a favorite candy, maybe my family, is different from what I understood once I'd fallen in love with a person; and a divorce and three subsequent relationships later, I have—*because* of those experiences—had to revise my understanding even further. Now I understand love through the lenses of loss and disappointment, but also through joys that have opened up my ideas of love's capacities.

I don't find any of these things particularly unbearable. Un-pin-downable, yes, but not unbearable. This was always true—I realize now—about my being queer also; I thought the answer to my confusion was being able to say "Yes, I'm a gay man," but no sooner had I said that than the question arose: "And what is a gay man?"

Understanding my queerness means I understand another facet of myself, but the facets, from what I can tell, are infinite—in their possibilities at least—and each new experience in a life shifts the light on those facets ever so slightly, which means they're newly shadowed also, which means, for a moment, we're disoriented, if not altogether lost, all over again.

I write in large part *toward* that lostness. It's in bewilderment that I come face to face with conundrum and, when I've written well, I emerge not having solved for X but having taken the measure of X, for now. Rather than erasing conundrum, I recalibrate my relationship to it, and in doing so, I feel something akin to stability, a stability that arises from pattern (patterns of thought, sound, image and feeling) and the meaningful, unpredictable interruption of pattern—which is all a poem is in the end, for me—a giving of form to shapelessness. The resulting stability isn't the stability of having my life make sense, but the stability of *feeling* like it makes sense, though if I had to parse that feeling, I couldn't—I wouldn't; the feeling itself is enough. (In this way, to have written a poem feels like the similarly unparseable closure that follows sex, but raised to a higher power.) That feeling, like the poem itself, is a shelter, for now, within the ever-changing, unpredictable weather of a life that continues until it won't, another conundrum I can't solve, I can only keep adjusting for it as it approaches, as I approach it.

I don't find the fact of death unbearable. I just find the impossibility of ever fully understanding that fact (we can know we're dying, but not that we're dead) a challenge to bear, or maybe more accurately, to know *how* to bear, which is maybe why, most days, most of us don't think about it. It's easier not to. It's easier not to write poems. It feels impossible—and maybe downright dangerous—to stop.

It's almost April here. In the garden, the perennials re-emerge in the configurations they were long ago planted in, they revive a pattern that each year, by the end of winter, I've almost forgotten. Then it's spring again. Very briefly, in spite of everything, the world again makes a kind of sense.

Warren Poland

Psychoanalyst, Writer

The Rest is Silence

My wife tells me that my epitaph should read, "NOW IT'S *YOUR* TURN TO TALK!"

This sentence was the result of a self-imposed challenge to see how brief a piece I could write that would still be long enough to sketch a person and an interaction. Sometimes an easy grader when it comes to myself, I at first felt content, feeling that my super-short communication succeeded in evoking both my characteristic verbosity and the fraying of patience this quality calls forth in my wife.

However, I rarely rest content with a first understanding. In actuality, the suggested epitaph arose not from my wife but from me. Yet had I not put the words in my wife's mouth, I would have been left with a sentence that sounded precious, one that appeared to have a smirk of self-admiration rather than a smile of interpersonal wit. The implicit dialogue between two people would disappear, leaving in its place the wearisome vanity of one congratulating himself on his own sense of humor.

If this were a first-person pronouncement, what would be even worse than the presence of my exposed vanity would be the absence of interpersonal interaction. Soliloquies that work, such as those created by Shakespeare, are not monologues but powerful dialogues between different parts of one person's mind. For writing to succeed there must be a give and take, at least an implicit conversation between a speaker and an emotionally responsive other. Lacking that is to be left with pure exposition, in which information may be transmitted but conversation absent.

Curiosity did not die after my one-sentence article grew to the length of what I have written so far. I next found myself turning from how I had written my exercise to concern for what was being said. I had to recognize more profound pressures underlying the already-noted superficial concerns of form.

It is much less common for an epitaph to speak the words of the dead person than for it to be a remembrance offered by those still

DOI: 10.4324/9781003516118-27

alive. My creating the inscription has, at least in fantasy, the quality of diluting—if not fully undoing—my demise. It is as if I were saying, "See, I can still have a conversation with you, the living. All right, perhaps I can no longer speak aloud for myself, but I can listen. Even though it may be lopsided, our conversation can continue, so death is not complete."

Of course, an irony of my single-sentence story is that my character, as the person who has died, is that of a long-winded talker. The imagined victory over death in my epitaph would thus carry with it the horrible personal punishment of my being confined to the hell of eternal listening without the power to speak. My imagined solution to dying etched on the tombstone is a dreadful failure. This being the case, I think I prefer the clarity of nonbeing to the mysteries of death.

In this note from me to you, dear reader, have I now done to you what I feared for myself? Have I turned you into the silent listener?

Now it's *your* turn to talk.

Permissions Line: Poland, Warren S. "The Rest Is Silence." *American Imago* 67:3 (2010), 451–452. © 2011 The Johns Hopkins University Press. Reprinted with permission of Johns Hopkins University Press.

Joshua Prager

Journalist, Author

When I was a little boy, I scratched three words into the side of my father's wooden bookcase: "DADDY HATES ME." They were the first words I remember writing, and I hoped for them to find their mark, to prompt an assurance of love or at least a reckoning. But my graffito went undiscovered. And by the time, a decade or so later, I left New Jersey for a gap year in Jerusalem, I wrote only for myself, chronicling, atop my twin bed in a mildewed stone dorm, life at eighteen.

My journal was less a stab at understanding than a log, a daily tally of push-ups and encounters and books. But there was rigor in the recapitulation, and some self-reflection, too; I had been away from home eight months when I wondered, in the wee hours of May 16, 1990, if I had the strength to be more religious than my parents.

Hours later, a runaway truck hit the rear of a minibus where I sat. My neck snapped back, two vertebrae broke and, within minutes, I could not move or speak, mouthing words that went unheard over the bustle of paramedics.

I was still quiet two weeks later when my right hand, calloused from disuse, began to buzz and twitch. I tried to move it. My index finger bent down, and I saw in its glorious little jerk a promise that I would write again. So I did; the whole of my right side had reinnervated when I graduated college, rose from my wheelchair and became a journalist, typing articles and then books with that same born-again finger.

I was not yet able to write of the catastrophe. "Wait without thought," wrote T.S. Eliot, "for you are not ready for thought: So the darkness shall be the light, and the stillness the dancing." And yet, as a journalist, I kept writing about lives that, like mine, had been changed in an instant—by the swing of a bat, the click of a shutter, an inheritance. And when, finally, I *was* ready to write of that singular moment that had redirected me, I returned to Jerusalem twenty years after the crash and found it at last articulable, the words coming forth as surely as the two glass pebbles that had emerged ten years before through a scar in my left arm.

DOI: 10.4324/9781003516118-28

On the page, the consequences of my broken neck were circumscribed. I could see them plain, see where the crash ended and I began. The writing was a catharsis, and I wished to rid myself of that other primordial hurt I had scratched as a boy into wood. But as with the crash, I was not yet ready to confront it. So, again, I wrote of other lives until, at last, I could write of my own. I am doing so now. My father is still alive. That is also reason to write.

Philip Schultz

Poet

Anger and Shame

Every strong creative impulse creates a cautionary reaction just as strong, and the more intimate and difficult our subject matter, the greater and more turbulent the reaction—is this why I so fear acknowledging in my work the harm and transgressions I may have caused, what might be revealed even in my successes? It's most certainly why I demand of myself some awareness of the process in which I'm so thoroughly engaged, why I interrogate myself at every step of the creative journey. It's also why I ask my students, before reading their work in class, to present preambles or statements in which they reiterate the criticism they heard the previous week, explain how they applied it, and then ask a question that best indicates what issue most preoccupied them during the writing. This question often proves the most challenging part and what I mostly hear back are general proclamations: whether there's a persona narrator present, or whether the mood or tone they were after is apparent. Few students ever ask the question so many writers find the most compelling and troubling: who may be hurt or offended by what they are writing. Joan Didion put this fear best in the preface to *Slouching Towards Bethlehem*: "*Writers are always selling somebody out.*" At some point every writer must deal with a similar question: Do we deserve satisfaction for causing pain to others, especially those we love?

Eugene O'Neill didn't allow what I consider his best play, *Long Day's Journey into Night*, which dealt with his most intimate and volatile feelings about his immediate family, to be published until twenty-five years after his death; Eudora Welty and Katherine Anne Porter waited until the end of their writing lives to deal with the potently complex situations and characters drawn from their personal histories in *Losing Battles* and *Ship of Fools*. To protect others and, ultimately, themselves, many writers meticulously disguise their characters and sometimes postpone essential material indefinitely. And in my experience, anger is the emotion that is

DOI: 10.4324/9781003516118-29

most often hidden behind this fear of self-incrimination, retribution, and insensitivity toward others. Anger and the shame it so often creates; the shame we feel for being angry at those we love. Maybe especially when anger is the appropriate response in a story or poem, it's seldom easily found; in fact, in otherwise finely orchestrated student work, it's often impossible to detect. And when I ask for the emotional truth in a scene or in lines of poetry, what I most often hear are excuses, apologies and static of all kinds. Yes, anger is what the majority of my students most stridently avoid and/or refuse to recognize in their work and sometimes in the work of others, even when its absence is glaringly obvious to me and many others.

One writer who ran away from home as a teenager and was forever trying to find her way back in her writing couldn't access the anger that made her leave home in the first place; another couldn't overcome the depths of her anger and shame in writing about a gay father who she felt had abandoned her as a child, and the ways in which this anger affected her eventual destruction of her family and herself as an adult; the union activist unafraid to take on tough factory bosses in standing up for workers' rights but unable to do the same against a domineering father; a writer so indoctrinated in spousal abandonments she stops writing just as she reaches the limits of her perceived allowance of indignation and success. Some, it would seem, would rather fail at what means most to them, their creative work, than confront painful truths, anger being, from my experience, the hardest to recognize and acknowledge. The imagination thrives on powerful emotions, and discovering what we're actually feeling under all the more stately and comfortable emotions we disguise them with can be a source of creative inspiration and thinking. Of its many forms and disguises, anger can be seen as reproach and instigation, a setting of boundaries and constraints, a system of checks and balances, a vow and a warning system so sophisticated and subtle we learn to both fear and appreciate its undeniable forecasts. And shame, what we so often feel in its wake, equally dominates and restricts our choice of subject matter and desire to confront shameful truths.

As Cioran said, "A negative habit is fruitful only so long as we exert ourselves to overcome it, adapt it to our needs." Writers learn to live with anxiety and exhilaration the way athletes learn to live with pain, yet so many of my students highlight a less menacing emotion at the expense of a more powerful one, which so disrupts their sense of equilibrium. And when anger's absence—that special rush of liquid fire—is obvious to everyone except the writer, I sometimes ask what the other students might feel if placed in the same position as the writer's narrator or character. Consensus of opinion provides not only verification but also the sense of solidarity and commiseration necessary to approach painful material. Even when camouflaged or diluted with satire and comedy, I'll point out, anger is prominent in many of the great works we study in craft class: Ginsberg's "Howl," Philip Larkin's "This Be the Verse," Yeats's "The Second Coming" and "Easter 1916" ("What is it but nightfall? /No, no, not night but death; /Wasn't it needless death after all?"), and Blake's "Morning" ("To Find the Western path/Right thro' the Gates of Wrath/I urge my way"); in Shakespeare's *Hamlet*, Ralph Ellison's *Invisible Man*, James Baldwin's *The Fire Next Time*, and Dante's revenge fantasies in *The Inferno*. Writers are in the business of divulging secrets, confessing to shames and regrets, but doing so often means using oneself as an example, as Keats does so powerfully in "Ode on a Grecian Urn": "Beauty is truth, truth beauty,—that is all/Ye know on earth, and all ye need to know."

Yes, Keats knew how emotionally expensive the exquisiteness of beauty and truth were to attain. Is this why it's not "possible to live in the bare present," as Martin Buber tells us in *I and Thou*, because the present would "consume" us if we didn't take precautions to defend ourselves against it? Why we can live only in "the bare past," where life can be organized, tolerated and enjoyed? Keats would've agreed with Buber that writing is a way of organizing the past well enough to find meaning in the present, where most of us want to live, even though it's where most of our pain and anger also reside. In that it makes us honest witnesses to our own acts of self-betrayal, suffering can be redemptive. And Keats had much to be angry about.

These lines are written on his tombstone in Rome:

> This grave contains all that was mortal of a young English poet who on his death-bed in the bitterness of his heart at the malicious power of his enemies desired these words to be engraved on his tombstone: Here lies One Whose Name was writ in Water.

He died of consumption at the age of twenty-five, having suffered scalding reviews of his work and perhaps, in his bitterness, desired the anonymity of being remembered only as an English poet to mock the way his critics viewed him. It's difficult to imagine such a self-regard for someone who wrote and left intact some of the most beautiful poetry ever written in English, but Keats obviously had his own shitbird to contend with, one that perhaps got in this last word. His acclaimed notion of negative capability, an idea that suggests that uncertainty and confusion can and will inspire, rather than oppose, creativity, isn't all that far removed from our notion that despair and self-contempt are opportunities for creative initiative. And nothing breeds uncertainty more than anger and the shame it so often creates. Nothing.

The black bird thrives in a state of permanent uncertainty, which it uses to anticipate and then smother creative excitement and appetite. Imagine then the force of will, the strength needed to inspire and sustain the refined lyrical resonance and creative intelligence that went into the creation of Keats's "Ode to a Nightingale," which so sensuously deals with that most tenuous, eternally resourceful state between sleep and waking, despite all the "bitterness of his heart."

> Forlorn! the very word is like a bell
> To toll me back from thee to my sole self!
> Adieu! the fancy cannot cheat so well
> As she is fam'd to do, deceiving elf.
> Adieu! adieu! thy plaintive anthem fades
> Past the near meadows, over the still stream,
> Up the hill-side; and now 'tis buried deep
> In the next valley-glades:
> Was it a vision, or a waking dream?
> Fled is that music:—Do I wake or sleep?

I once became incensed while visiting the grave of a friend whose encouragement and criticism helped me write my book of poems *Failure*. Though I'd always loved the Baudelaire quote friends had put on his gravestone—*The dispersion and reconstitution of the self. /That's the whole story*—I now saw it as blatantly obscure and personally insulting. Yes, epitaph as slander. Why would he, so gifted, wise and assiduous about all matters literary, want such an emblem to represent him for eternity? And how had I allowed it? I felt overcome with remorse and chagrin.

My friend had died abruptly of cancer shortly before my book was published and though I couldn't acknowledge it, I was left feeling abandoned and betrayed and, yes, angry. And having buried the anger along with the shame it created, I wasn't able to complete an elegy I'd spent years trying to write for him. Without realizing it, I'd come there that morning begging for inspiration and, perhaps, permission to finish my poem for him. And now, having erupted in anger for no real reason I could understand, I was overcome with shame and bewilderment, and began weeping. What sort of wretched person was I to be angry at a dear friend for dying two weeks before his fifty-second birthday? And just as suddenly as it'd erupted, the anger was gone, and these lines came:

> I've forgiven you, finally,
> for not living to see the book you helped me write
> get published. Only now do I understand that
> it's not the resentment I regret, it's the shame.

Lines that opened up into my elegy, "Welcome to the Springs," for my friend Robert Long. Anger, and the shame it caused, had blocked not only the grief but the forgiveness I was seeking. And then, not long after I finished this poem, I began wondering if there wasn't another way of helping my students overcome their own fears and misgivings. To confront in this same way emotions so difficult to even recognize. Yes, the same ominous emotions and the gravitational forces they created around them to repel further inspection seemed to discourage so many from even recognizing potentially powerful subject matter; once again, the shitbird's most perverse and persuasive weapon its invisibility. If you can't recognize your desire to deal with material that so often proves to be inspiring, you most certainly can't find the will to do so.

Occasionally, when suggesting to someone what might be hidden behind a strand of dialogue, an abbreviated scene and stanza, stuttering, coughing or squirming erupts. Whatever is causing such upset, I may then suggest, might be seen as an opportunity to find an "I" or "We" or "You" brave, tolerant, and opinionated enough to confront the origins of their discontent. That inside their assembly of orchestrated personalities, the great democracy of voices we carry around within us, an "I" exists abundant enough to inhabit what Walt Whitman believed to be his own strength of vision: "I will effuse egotism and show it underlying all, and I will be the bard of personality. . . . And that all things of the universe are perfect miracles, each as profound as any." Yes, indeed, "the bard of personality" great enough to overcome all our foolishness and vain posturing, all the evidence of our greed and stupidity, so we might believe our one small voice is "as profound as any."

Left unexpressed, anger and its attendant passion, shame, engender only futility and failure. Without first realizing and then submitting to our fears and inadequacies, our ever-subservient and fragile vulnerability, there can be no catharsis, and thus, no poetry.

Permissions Line, UK: "Anger and Shame" from *Comforts of the Abyss* by Philip Schultz. Copyright © 2024 by Philip Schultz. Reprinted by permission of Georges Borchardt, Inc. on behalf of the author. All rights reserved.

Permissions Line, US: "Anger and Shame," from COMFORTS OF THE ABYSS: THE ART OF PERSONA WRITING by Philip Schultz. Copyright © 2022 by Philip Schultz. Used by permission of W. W. Norton & Company, Inc.

Michael Slevin

Psychotherapist, Writer, Editor

Writing, Reporting and Working-Through

Laid up in bed, pelvis fractured, I put pencil to paper. I am six.

From stone to stone, memory to memory, I leap across the River of Forgetfulness. I remember, I repeat, I work-through.

As the bone knits, my mother teaches me to spell, the shadowy figure of my father looming.

So began my career as a writer.

#

My father was a reporter. A newspaper reporter. The fancy word today is "journalist." And today, journalism is a fancy career—a professional career, even. But after the War—the Second World War, that is—when my father started out, news was still tinged by the raw era of Ben Hecht's *Front Page*, and reporting was not the career his assimilating Jewish parents had hoped for.

I knew him as a reporter. I even read words he had written in his newspaper, *The New York Herald Tribune*, after school, sitting at the round table in our kitchen as my mother fixed dinner. But for the hard news of his Washington economic reporting? I pulled the split-page, Jimmy Breslin, for the hard-nosed stories reported from the street.

Blood relatives became reporters. Even *I* pulled a check from *The Washington Post*, *Congressional Quarterly*, *The Chronicle of Higher Education*. Some people, including my second analyst, tied my aspirations to "the family business." In my gut, I denied shares in any such entity.

Writers.

#

DOI: 10.4324/9781003516118-30

It is sometimes said writers have but one story; they repeat it over and over, themes and variations. So here, as I begin, is the story of family traumas which shaped my life, with this rock-bottom variation: "How it is I came to write," remembered, repeated and, by the end of the essay, worked-through, I hope, more than before. The relationship with my father was condensed in episodes at two critical stages of my life: one when I was a toddler, asserting autonomy; the other at age six.

As a toddler, I fell from a second-story window. Late that afternoon, brought to a city hospital. Bright lights, a whirring sound as they looked inside my head. Left alone for overnight observation; the terror of abandonment. My parents must have harbored great shame and guilt as they kept secret that I had fallen. My own memories hidden in dreams, unrecognized. My father told me, twenty years later, that he and my grandmother came for me in the morning. He told me I squirmed down from his arms and marched out on my own. I didn't trust my father.

The second crisis came at age six. As I built a tower in a sandpile, a neighbor backed into me with her car, fracturing my pelvis. I remember lying on my back on the exam table in the emergency room, the doctor with large shears cutting off my shorts.

There was an insurance settlement, not much, for pain and suffering. Years later, I remembered word for word an argument my parents had over the settlement. My father thought the proposed amount insufficient, wanted to counter it. My mother's instinct was to protect her careless friend, not cause *her* more pain. Abandoned again.

My mother was present, though, in a different way. Concretely, it was her blanket box I climbed up on to reach the window ledge I fell from. In my late teens, I dreamed I had fallen from a great height; scrambling, then, up a yellow brick wall, apartment windows dark, unable to get all the way back up.

My mother was present as my fractured pelvis healed. There is evidence. I hold the school report card. The first square for a handwritten evaluation is blank. I see my attendance was broken off just days after first clambering up the steps of a school bus, leaving behind the playground of summer. Instead, injured, confined to bed, I had to depend on my mother for bodily functions—and for lessons. By mid-October she had taught me first grade. She had returned to my life, now a confused blur of Eros, anger, guilt and shame. My schooling and emotional growth were soon paralyzed.

My mother was also a refuge where my murderous rage went underground. My father was often angry at me. His criticism felt relentless, and repeatedly I offered myself up. At the beach once, in my early twenties, I spent half an hour alone on a second level deck thinking about, turning over, the word "so." Excited, I came in to tell him of my explorations. He was curtly dismissive: "The word 'so' means '*so*.' Period."

#

In the spring of 2015, I went to work in the emergency department of an urban community hospital. My title: Psychiatric Evaluator. My job: interview children, adolescents and adults in psychological crises to determine if they were a danger to themselves or others, whether they could go home or would require admission to a psychiatric inpatient unit. Later, I would write, as an essay for a journal and book collection:

> As I learned the ropes, I worked with restless anxiety. So much at stake for my patients, so much dread I might be mistaken. It took three years for the needed knowledge to distill, for me to be comfortable making those decisions.

A person in the ER in psychological crisis is suffering acutely. While the Evaluator's essential task is to protect life, within the stillness of an interview there is opportunity to connect, to understand, to heal. I get a history, aware of its roots in family relationships, living circumstances, developmental history and intrapsychic conflict, but focused on the immediate crisis. I listen, staying alert to catch my stream of memories, my biases, cultural history and personal traumas, how they give insight or misdirect. I float above.

A pediatric emergency room bustles with energy, at times with noise; the lights are bright; sometimes infants cry, or a rambunctious child is hard to contain. One evening, as I walked over to see a patient, I suddenly remembered the two times as a young child I had been treated for physical trauma in hospital emergency rooms. In that moment, I understood my terror; I was enacting a childhood wish to know what the doctors thought was going on inside my head: to get home to my mother, to turn back the clock, to obliterate the fall and all that followed. I was healing myself.

Writing about my ER patients also heals.

#

In 2018, I walked over to the round table in our kitchen alcove. With pen and paper I sat down to write: "Of Being and Becoming: Psychoanalysis, Race, and Class in an Urban ER."

My opening words: "Heal thyself."

Then came: "Know thyself."

Next, I described the place, the purpose:

> I work in the emergency room of an urban hospital, evaluating people in psychological crisis. Are they a danger to themselves or others? Are they suicidal? Homicidal? Are they safe?

Then I could drop into my first case vignette.

A middle-school African American girl I worked with told me about her father with a pain she could not numb. He had been shot in the head and killed when she was five, an age when little girls have very intense feelings for their fathers. Her mother remarried. A few years later, her stepfather was stabbed to death. When I saw her in the ER, she was severely depressed. I felt her anguish in my gut; a door had cracked open to a world barely touched by crime-blotter newspaper stories tinged with race. She had opened the door to her sadness; for me, a bucket plunged into a deep well. Like this young girl, backed into her pillows, who twice had had fathers ripped from her life, I had feelings of profound isolation and father abandonment.

Yet, although I shared in her world, I was not part of it.

#

To tell our stories requires trust. I was constantly navigating trust in the emergency room to create a safe place for a story to be told, for work to be done. As I write this essay on becoming a writer, I find myself in pain remembering words recently spoken to me. My wife, who is an African American psychoanalyst and psychiatrist, once told me that few Black people coming to an ER in urgent psychological crisis would trust a white therapist. Shaken and confused, I resisted with a plaintive request for reassurance: I had been worthy of trust. Hadn't I made emotionally rich connections with many African American patients and their families? One nurse I told goodbye to after I resigned had said simply, "Your patients will miss you."

Yet, the memory of one patient presses forward. Here's what I had written in 2018:

> At other times, distrust is palpable. A six-year-old African American boy sat on the white sheet of his hospital bed, feet dangling; he stared directly at me. His eyes, black, round and frightened, shielded by street smarts beyond his years, dared me, "You want to find me out? I don't want to be here; I will tell you nothing that'll keep me here."

It took at least a couple of hours at the round table to write those sentences. Resistance to knowing his degree of distrust had barred access to emotionally precise memories. I struggled to bring his face into focus, to distill the experience his eyes told, to find words for what had happened between us. For all that, did I ever truly *get* the experience my African American patients had of being in crisis, dependent on white pediatric ER professional staff? That is, had I ever truly brought into focus and distilled my experience as a white clinician on the upside of structural racism seeking to help African Americans on the downside? No. I had not.

#

One day, as I worked on this essay, my wife and I were taking care of our grandchildren: two boys, twenty months and three years old. The year before, coming home from a weekend outing, their car had been rear-ended at high speed. Fortunately, no one was hurt. But on this day, the older boy and I, on his initiative, were playing an intense game of "Crash!"

A dream two nights later told me the child was not the only one working on his trauma. In the dream, construction, a tall building; a crane of many stories. For a moment, a hillside, an overlook, still. Abruptly, the tower: I am on its outside, hold tight to its interior platform moving down. The dream morphs: I stand on the platform, then fade: there, a girl, five years old, reaching the ground. A clutch of journalists mills about. Around a turn, to a distance, I sit comfortably on my haunches. The girl, with her mother now, alone. I watch. Suddenly: the girl runs from her mother, shrieking with joy, into my arms. I tell her Freud has written a paper about this: "It is called 'The Uncanny,'" I say, and "I will explain it to you."

In the dream, I become the father I needed. As I wrote the original essay, and now this essay about writing the original paper, I come closer to knowing the Writer I need to be.

Rita Dove

Poet

"Driven to write" carries with it the suggestion that one is being coerced into an undesirable situation, like cattle shunted to slaughter—along with the implication that there are forces beyond one's control operating behind the scenes, just as windswept leaves or snow drifts are helpless to direct their path or impact their fate. But for me, this could not be further from the truth: I yearn to be in a constant state of flight, tumbling along an unexplored trail just to discover where it will deposit me.

Of course, there were other paths to bliss I might have followed. My love affair with music—making it, charting it, reveling in the interstices of melody, harmony, counterpoint—began at approximately the same age as my first serious forays into writing. I was around ten years old when I first wallowed in the meaty measures of Shakespeare, then tried my hand at scoring noun-verb-adjective along the rolling twists and breaks of syntax, venturing to craft my own poems whenever I wasn't practicing my cello. In the end, however, the primary pleasures of writing, of original composition, won out over the secondary joys of instrumental interpretation; I felt privileged to have found this entry into the mysterious enterprise of creation. That these human grunts and hisses and snarls, these clicks and slithers and intoned gasps could coalesce to compile a grocery list or tell a joke, all the way to the point of articulating the complex, barely speakable apprehensions our flesh is heir to—the wonders of language already struck me dumb (what a jewel of an oxymoron!) when I was a child, and have never left me.

One of my early mentors once declared that writing is an exuberant discipline, as much ecstasy as profession. Perhaps the "driven" part only pertains when I am struggling with a particular piece of language, which of course happens, and should happen, in every poem I write—successful or not. But if, during the process, there is no passage which challenges all my faculties and drives me near to despair with its orneriness, I don't see how the poem that emerges could be remotely interesting to anyone else.

DOI: 10.4324/9781003516118-31

I love to write. I hate to write. I've been involved in this enterprise—call it a vocation or a mission; I can't think of it as anything but *Who I Am*—for so long, it's tempting to say it's just what I do, or it's how I've organized my days and nights, or that it's too late to reconsider and take a different tack. But the real truth is that I wouldn't turn back if given every chance in the world. That frustration fizzling to dead ends or breaking into delight, the oscillations of radiance and terror—I adore the whole roller coaster ride.

3

Evidence and Experiences

Ellen Pinsky and Michael Slevin

Ellen Pinsky

Teacher, Psychoanalyst

Three Propositions About Writing

I *hate* writing. Writing is hell. Or, let me cast that more moderately: Writing is difficult for me and for many people I know, including professional writers. Why?

Writing isn't natural. It's work, and—often enough—frustrating work, full of anxiety, doubt, false starts, dead ends. A friend who is a writer once quipped: "There are two activities for the writer, and both are agony: one is called 'writing,' the other 'not-writing.' There's a brief happy period in between called 'having written.'"

Why, then, does anyone do it? Sometimes, it's required; in many professions, one has to write to get a degree or a credential. But why do sociologists, poets, essayists, novelists, journalists write? Why do comedy writers write? Among many answers (including money, or the wish for it), one might be: "I really don't know why, I just *need* to write." But as a psychoanalyst, do I need (credential requirements aside) to write? How have I understood my own struggle with writing?

Writing is thinking, and thinking has to include discomfort. There's a striving for something. Every human being's first thought, according to Freud, is unpleasant, forced on us by an unsatisfying reality. In his early essay "Formulations on the Two Principles of Mental Functioning," Freud elaborates a sequence: the baby is distressed; it conjures a presence, what's wished for but absent—feeding, say, or comfort. Freud calls this mental activity the "attempt at satisfaction by means of hallucination." Relief, however, doesn't always come, and with that disappointment, the "psychical apparatus" (here Freud means the baby) has to "form a conception of the real circumstances in the external world and to endeavor to make a real alteration in them." The baby's attention turns from inside to outside; and in this shift, thinking—or striving—begins, along with separation from the mother.

DOI: 10.4324/9781003516118-33

Perhaps I exaggerate the misery of writing, as did Freud, who acknowledged that his schematic terms merely provide a useful "fiction." But despite the abstract polysyllabic language, this useful fiction about the baby's developing mind helps me understand the difficulty and pain of writing.

I'll offer three propositions about writing.

Proposition One: Writing is hard work. Some may tell you, if you write well, writing is easy: good writing is inspired, it spills out, it *flows* like a river. Just let your muse speak, and go with the flow . . . No. It's not like a river. It does not flow. It's more like being a beaver in the river: building a dam, gnawing, sawing, placing and re-placing branches— deploying sharp teeth, muscular tail, chewing and thwacking away. Writers resemble large, nocturnal, semi-aquatic rodents.

The benign myth of "inspired flow" disrespects the real work of making sentences that actually say something. The writer Javier Marias, in the foreword to a collection of his stories, *When I Was Mortal*, tells the reader that, of the twelve stories in the book, eleven were commissioned, their lengths set by others. Marias writes:

> It is perhaps worth reminding those sentimental purists who believe that, in order to sit down in front of a typewriter, you have to experience grandiose feelings such as a creative 'need' or 'impulse,' which are always 'spontaneous' or terribly intense, that the majority of the sublime works of art produced over the centuries—especially in painting or music—were the result of commissions or of even more prosaic or servile stimuli.

I admit Marias also notes: "I can only write something if I'm enjoying myself, and I can only enjoy myself if I find the project interesting . . . [N]one of these stories would have been written if I had felt no interest in them." Or, as George Orwell puts it in his essential essay "Why I Write," "I could not do the work of writing . . . if it were not also an aesthetic experience." From this we can extract further tips: pleasure is involved. For Orwell, there's pleasure in the "perception of beauty in the external world, or . . . in words and their right arrangement." Marias can only write the story if he feels interest. And he links writing, enjoyment and interest. We might wonder why. What does it mean "to feel interest?"

That takes me to Proposition Two: The most important things about writing are the same for all writing. Before I became a psychoanalyst, I was a middle school English teacher for many years. How to get eleven- and twelve-year-olds to say something, to say *anything*, about whatever they were reading?

One day I found a magic word, a verb: to notice. "What do you notice?" I asked, nothing more. Silence at first, then a wisecrack or two. But it was a question, and a word, the children were willing to play with and, over time, take greater risks to answer. "What do you notice?" helped them locate interest, create focus, find enjoyment. Sometimes the act of noticing helped them like a poem or story better. And as writers, they also relaxed, trusting they could find something to say—they had thoughts!

Of course it's not that simple. But here's the point: the problem most of us face in writing isn't simply techniques of writing. The problem is awareness, attention, focus, interest, noticing: can you give yourself to what you notice?

By "give yourself" I don't mean going with the flow, but embracing the truth that one is often thinking when it doesn't feel like thinking. Whatever you catch hold of, it's *about* something; it's a flag, a marker, and offers a start. When I was required to write about the clinical work with one of my patients, I remember feeling stymied, blocked—the usual. But in some random moment, what came to mind was a familiar scene I had noticed: I saw the young man breeze into the room, talking rapidly with a cozy, manipulative good cheer that took my breath away, effectively silencing me. That scene contained the story of the treatment, and I began my written account with it.

I expect the reader has noticed my words: "what came to mind." Here, I'm suggesting that the anxiety of writing is not unlike the anxiety of the associative process itself. What will one say? What will come up? What will float in? And perhaps it's true enough that, just as talking is the cure, so too is the writing.

The cure for what? That takes me to the Third Proposition: Writing is a process of mourning and entails loss—in Freud's language, "working-through." Much could be said about different forms of writing. Some will insist that describing the work with my patient is a completely different task than other kinds of writing: not the same as writing a poem, a theoretical essay, a legal brief or a comic riff for Stephen Colbert. I disagree. Writing always tells a story.

What is a story? Forget chronology—a story is not a chronological regurgitation. When Freud describes his toddler grandson repeatedly tossing his toy, a wooden spool on a string, over the side of his cot, "Fort," and pulling it back, "Da!", not only is that the first recorded psychoanalytic infant observation, but it is also a story: the story of the baby's loss ("fort") and wished-for retrieval ("da"); mother goes away, mother returns. Tireless, patient, like the beaver building the dam, back and forth, over and over, the little boy endures his pain by *making* something—it is an aesthetic experience. The game, playing "gone," (says Freud in *Beyond the Pleasure Principle*), is the child's "great cultural achievement."

There's an additional poignancy to the nursery scene: Freud first observes the toddler's game in 1915 but writes the narrative five years later, when the child is not quite six. The boy's mother has recently died. That mother is Freud's daughter Sophie, twenty-six years old and pregnant when she dies of influenza. Whose imagination is at work here, overcoming pain? Who's playing "gone," whose grief are we witnessing in the writer's description of the little boy's game? In the shadows, there's something else the grandfather and writer knows: this particular, actual child who is playing at tossing the reel/mother away will in 1920, at age five, lose that mother forever.

All development happens against the backdrop of loss. In giving up the Eden of omnipotence, a recurring surrender that never ends until the final loss, Freud's toddler finds comfort. The game tells a story of mastery, of aggression, of vengeance and creative problem-solving. The wooden spool, like the mother, is gone, and then returns, saying, in effect, "Da! I am here!" But even more important, the boy who creates the drama is also saying, "I am here: *I* did this, I'm the one who *made* it!" In this game, there's never a moment of doubt who controls that wooden spool! The boy stages a "joyful return," and Freud adds another motive—the turning of passive to active, as if, with comedy and delight, he speaks the child's defiance: *"All right then, go away! I don't need you. I'm sending you away myself."* There's the additional satisfaction of the child's revenge: he throws her away. In repeating the represented experience of abandonment and return, he's like a poet finding a form, and like his essayist grandfather, making something and working through his grief—the little boy is the choreographer of loss.

Elsewhere, Freud says:

> Writing was in its origin the voice of an absent person, and the dwelling-house was a substitute for the mother's womb, the first lodging, for which in all likelihood man still longs, and in which he was safe and felt at ease.

In other words, "fort-da."

On these terms, all writing—all successful or "true" writing—is a form of working-through; a grieving process. So of course it's hard. When the psychoanalyst-writer tells the story of an intimacy built over time with a suffering, striving person who has come for help, she is re-connecting as well as saying good-bye, separating herself out as well as rejoining. The narration creates a bond while it sets free both herself and the patient.

If we think of both narrative and analytic work as a process of mourning, we may understand and appreciate better the reality of the difficulty and of the reward. Maybe what I have been telling here is my own story of striving: a teacher of reading and writing who became a psychoanalyst, and is working to become a writer.

I began with the three words: "I hate writing." It's pure hell writing about how much I hate writing about hating writing. Who am I writing this for? Is it to encourage and comfort *you*? Or is it to encourage and comfort me? Either way, having begun with three words, I'll end with three: get to work!

Adam Phillips

Psychoanalyst, Writer

Psychoanalysis in Writing

When we write about psychoanalysis, what do we imagine we are writing about? There are, at one end, the manuals of psychoanalytic theory and technique written in a familiar and accessible vocabulary, and at the other end there are vivid, evocative and enigmatic clinical vignettes. Or, there are innovatory theoretical proposals which seem to require a new vocabulary, a less predictable idiom. Efforts to consolidate theory and practice attempt to embrace this entire range, sometimes with the goal of unsettling some assumed consensus.

If psychoanalysis, in any of its various versions, is a science—or akin to one—it is, in Thomas Kuhn's language, an ongoing set of more or less prescribed experiments, unless or until there is what Kuhn calls a paradigm shift, after which we do different kinds of experiments. We are, then, in search of tentative hypotheses that are potentially falsifiable as a foundation for the discipline: guidelines or blueprints for theory and practice. In psychoanalysis, these hypotheses are about so-called human nature. Psychoanalysis, that is to say, is not deemed to be local knowledge; as is the way with science, it has universalizing ambitions.

In this crude account of a scientific psychoanalysis, we get better and better at describing human nature, and at diagnosing and treating what people are suffering from. In this by now traditional myth of progress—psychoanalysis as a branch of medicine—we become increasingly efficient at alleviating the difficulties people have in living. This medical model requires the practicing analyst to keep up with the research, and to use it. The scientifically inclined (or tempted) analyst is always mindful that the supposed, aspired-to objectivity has ethical implications.

The analyst who doesn't want to be a scientist, or who doesn't only want to be a scientist, undertakes a much more ambiguous project in writing about psychoanalysis. When she is not confirming or disconfirming

DOI: 10.4324/9781003516118-34

the available theory and practice, she may be doing something in her writing that is either less clear or not entirely formulatable. She may in some sense, in the words of the critic R.P. Blackmur, be "adding to the stock of available reality"—or to the stock of available psychoanalytic reality—but she may not quite know what she is adding or how, if at all, what she is adding can be useful for herself, or for anyone beyond herself. The psychoanalytic writer runs the risk of falling out of the language of psychoanalysis. She can begin to sound like someone writing fiction or poetry or philosophy. It may not always be clear when what is being written is psychoanalysis, or what it is to write unalloyed psychoanalysis.

At what point does the psychoanalytically informed reader think, "This is not psychoanalysis" about any given piece of writing? At such moments, the criteria for recognizing psychoanalytic writing may be taken to be patent, agreed upon and consciously acknowledged. When I am thinking, "This is not psychoanalysis" because it is fiction, or ideology, or cognitive psychology, or theology, or sociology, or moral theory, or delirium or delusion, I am aligning myself with a group of people who know what psychoanalysis is, and what it involves. As precedent, of course, there is the famous moment when Freud, in his *Studies on Hysteria*, remarks that his case-histories sound like short stories. The reader can then wonder: "and what's wrong with that?"—and everything depends on the answer to the question.

When we are not writing psychoanalysis, or about psychoanalysis, more or less under the aegis of science, we don't really know what we are doing—other, that is, than possibly contributing to the dream-day of the reader. Or, more simply, engaging his or her attention and interest. That is to say, we can write psychoanalysis for the pragmatist, for the dreamer or for both. And by the same token, we can write psychoanalysis as pragmatists and/or as dreamers. The pragmatist, broadly speaking, knows how he wants his writing to be used—he wants it to persuade someone of something—and that it can be used and therefore shared (it can be applied). The dreamer can predict nothing about the effect of his writing, and may not want to. The pragmatist writes with intent, the dreamer writes in hope—in hopeful and unpredictable anticipation. The pragmatist says, "this is what it should be like for us"; the dreamer says, "this is what it's like for me."

The psychoanalytic writer, or the writer of psychoanalysis—clearly not always the same thing—might wonder, then, what they want from the writing of psychoanalysis, just as the reader of psychoanalysis may wonder whether she wants to be informed or to be provoked, to be instructed or to dream. The function of language, Lacan once remarked, is not only to inform but also to evoke. When psychoanalytic writing is more evocative than informative, what is it doing for psychoanalysis? To what is it contributing?

Once psychoanalytic writing disidentifies itself from science, and ceases to be propaganda, it has a less palpable design on the reader. The writer can recover her unconscious intentions. She can write something other than—something as well as—what she had intended to write. Something one might have thought that the psychoanalytic writer would be, in the nature of the psychoanalytic pursuit, committed to. As I am.

Rowan Ricardo Phillips

Poet

On "The Question"

The origin story of a poet is more a myth than anything else. But I'm uneasy with the moniker of "poet": it often feels a distant and honorific sobriquet that only means what it's intended to mean in one moment—poets are poets when writing poetry; when they're not writing poetry they are not.

We are first taught as children to understand the world through rhythm. Even the alphabet, with which we form all our words, comes to us as song. The urge toward poetry is inherent in our initial understanding of the world, it is the baseline of our being. But as we mature, the world of prose and its accompanying socializing imperatives (statements do not sing, reasons do not rhyme, answers do not ask) forces that urge to recede deep within us. Those who write poetry have maintained their access to this urge; but this urge is something that we all have.

I think of this when I'm asked, as I am frequently, the question which begins my poem "The Question." It comes up all the time: "When did you know you wanted to become a poet?" It's a performative thing, both for the questioner and the recipient of the question; a moment in which we're supposed to bask in the recollection of turning desire into transformation, where one who did not have the power of poetry turns into someone who does.

Unwittingly, in this moment everyone plays their role, though I doubt anyone involved believes in the role they're playing. "I knew I wanted to become a poet after reading this one poem that I loved" or "I knew I wanted to become a poet after hearing a wolf in the distance howl at the moon and looking up and seeing no moon in the sky" or "I knew I wanted to become a poet because my mother used to recite poems to me and nothing else has ever seemed so beautiful." What does the questioner do with any of these answers? Do they perform a test run themselves? Or have they simply gotten to know a little more about the poet?

DOI: 10.4324/9781003516118-35

Poets are, of course, utterly unreliable narrators, especially when it comes to their lives as poets—as they should be. Plato was right about us. I find these little boxes of narratives of being and becoming that we try to cram poetry into curious and archetypal. This may be why "The Question" is a sonnet—an archetypal little box for the curious.

Poetry is not the question we ask in public, but the question that remains with you afterward in private. That beautiful, needful thing that is "part of the poem, /The part where it all comes together, and, /Having come together, finally sings."

THE QUESTION

When did you know you wanted to become
A poet? No one believes this question.
No one listens for the answer. It's one
Of those habits of people forced to live
Together on a spinning rock, the pale
Blue dot a wince in the wide attention
The dying light seeks out from ice giants
Dull and firm in the dark, under polite
Lights, midst rows and rows of people who ask
When and why about poetry, of she
Who forgets to ask something that was,
I realize later, part of the poem,
The part where it all comes together, and,
Having come together, finally sings.

Permissions Line, UK: Rowan Ricardo Phillips, "The Question" from *Living Weapon*. Copyright © 2021 by Rowan Ricardo Phillips. Reprinted with the permission of Faber and Faber Ltd.

Permissions Line, US: "The Question" from LIVING WEAPON by Rowan Ricardo Phillips. Copyright © 2018 by Rowan Ricardo Phillips. Reprinted by permission of Farrar, Straus and Giroux. All rights reserved.

Rachel Dillon

Poet, Editor, Teacher

Benevolent Ghosts

As a child, I kept everything: check-out receipts from the library, old Red Sox tickets, school valentines from classmates I barely knew, business cards from every bagel shop I ever visited.

For my eighth birthday, I asked for a Polaroid camera. There were plenty of digital options, but I wanted immediate photos that I could hold, date and keep in a box.

For my ninth birthday, I asked for a label maker so I could Dewey Decimal my collection of books into a "real" library, the highlights of which included all the *Ramona and Beezus* books and Charles Schulz's complete *Peanuts* collection.

I was a neurotic, sensitive child—prerequisites for becoming a poet, maybe. I was scared to forget anything. I was also scared of being forgotten.

My earliest writing projects took the form of letters to the family who would live in our home after my family left. I didn't know, of course, who this family might be, but I loved the idea of them discovering my messages from the past. I magic-markered long reports of my daily life on Bartlett Ave and hid them under the dusty red and blue flagstones threading through the backyard.

My mother, who always encouraged my strange little projects, warned me that my letters would be lost to the elements. So, together, we unearthed and wrapped each letter in elaborate layers of tape, tinfoil, and Ziploc bags before burying them again. After a summer rainstorm proved that our protective measures weren't enough, I took a more traditional approach: I began journaling in a small purple book the size of my palm. I wrote until each page was dappled with ballpoint imprints, then hid the journal behind the radiator in my bedroom for someone to find.

My family moved out of Bartlett Ave earlier than planned, shortly after I'd begun middle school and long after I forgot that journal. Years later, a

DOI: 10.4324/9781003516118-36

woman who had moved into our old house mailed us the little journal with a note: "Found this while replacing the heating system. I promise I didn't read it!" I didn't believe her—who wouldn't read a mysterious journal, and how else would she know where to send it?

The journal had been hidden for close to ten years. When I re-read it as a teenager, I was struck by the melodramatic voice I'd adopted (likely influenced by Anne Frank's diary and the tragedy of the Romanovs, two moments in history I was obsessed with as a kid). While the words felt unfamiliar, reading them transported me to the moments I spent writing: sitting on the back patio hunched over my journal, a Hoodsie cup melting beside me, the sounds of crickets and passing cars. My childhood self was waving to me, helping me remember the texture of what my life was once like.

A poet friend told me that our brains are designed to forget more than they retain. It's the best way we can make space for new memories. It frightens me still, how many small moments I've forgotten, how many I'll soon forget. Writing, reading and re-writing pull me back towards those days and selves I feel disconnected from. It's the closest proof I have of the existence of ghosts.

The way I feel when I draft a poem is how I imagine someone might feel when they've entered a state of meditation. It's shocking how quickly I lose track of time—how elements of the sacred, the Rabbis of my childhood, wander onto the page—how memories circle like benevolent ghosts. The American modernist painter and poet Marsden Hartley titled his autobiography *Somehow a Past*; to me, this sums it up. Somehow, as I write, my mind surprises me and links me to a past, again and again. And it's not only the words themselves—when I revisit a poem or revise a draft, I can usually recall exactly where I was sitting when I first wrote it. The poem allows me to capture memories on the page as well as the moment in my life when it was written.

I recently found an old folder of poem scraps I'd written as an undergraduate. At first, it was alarming to revisit. Sure, I could see how my writing had improved since then, but the ideas, the anxieties, the preoccupations were the same as those I write about now. Had I not changed at all over the last decade? Hadn't I grown? Become braver?

I was upset by this lack of growth, but later found comfort in the similarities; the kinship I felt with my former self. My daily life as a student was different, yet my heart, my brain—so much is still the same. I texted my husband: "Everyone should have this." By "this," I meant direct access to a former self. The ability to transcend time and space through writing, and to reconnect, somehow, to a particular past.

I still hold on to ephemera: tickets, receipts, sticky notes. I tuck them between the pages of whatever book I'm reading at that moment, or old books on my shelves. Many of those books still sport Dewey Decimal numbers and genres on their spines, the labels sun-faded and peeling.

I like to imagine some future grandchild of mine poring over my dusty collection of books, just as my mother and I spent hours finding treasures in my grandmother's closet after her death. I like to think of that grandchild opening my copy of Elsa Morante's *History* and discovering an espresso ring on page 535 from the summer I spent in Italy, or flipping through my graduate school annotations of Brigit Pegeen Kelly's *Song*. Ghosts waving from the page.

Anne Adelman

Psychoanalyst, Writer, Editor

In my parents' typewriter store, writing was a physical, breathing, noisy experience. Paper crinkling, rollers cogwheeling softly, carriages leveraged into place. Fingers tapping keys were set against the pulse of metal striking platens, the ding at the end of the line, the zip of the carriage readied to begin the next. Each machine had its own rhythm, a unique touch beneath the hand, a melody that melded with one's thoughts and formed into words on a blank page.

The cramped store bustled. Writers entered the space in front of the counter clutching their machines tightly to their chests, reluctant to spend even an hour without their typewriters. From a small stool beside my father, I watched while his customers hovered anxiously. My father would take out a tool and carefully, lovingly prod the keys, looking for the source of a loose "m" or a jumpy "k." As the writers waited, they typed words on random machines propped open on the countertop, a sheet of paper already slipped into the carriage waiting for their eager fingers. "The quick brown fox" transformed into a poem, a musing about the weather, an ode to my father the "typewriter magician" or the impatient "grrrrrrrrrr" of a writer waiting for his machine to be restored. When the workday ended, I'd collect these scraps, words flung onto a page that captured a moment in time, a stray idea, a thought that appeared and vanished just as quickly.

My home was filled with the language of immigrants and refugees. In this universe of words, though, it was the written ones that offered refuge. In a world out of sync with that of my peers, writing warmed me. My parents gave me a typewriter with a broken case, left behind by a customer and sitting forlornly in the back of the store. I would sit outside in the sun, wrapped in a quilt, typing the words that flowed into my head. I spent hours making up stories set in faraway places that I half-thought were true. I lost myself in the characters, imagining places and people for whom anything was possible. Magical,

DOI: 10.4324/9781003516118-37

fantastical, they bounded past the constraints of ordinary life. Writing transported me.

My childhood's type-scribbling gave way to aching adolescent poetry that grappled with the beauty and terror of solitude. With nothing but books around me, I would write outdoors on cool autumn days, in the light of the waning sun. But I lacked perspective, experience and guidance; I was too vulnerable to rejection, criticism or suggestion. My words began to falter, my freedom with ideas grew restricted and I became saddled with self-doubt. I could not endure having my stories, securely bound and packed into earnest-looking manila envelopes, turned away with indifference by the editors I entreated. Having revealed myself without restraint and been rejected, I was overtaken with shame and wanted to pull back. Before I was through college, I shut down any aspiration of a writing career. I turned to studying the life of the mind rather than contriving it in fiction.

Soon after, the days I knew in my parents' typewriter store came to a slow, rumbling stop. A number of events had converged: the word processor and personal computer emerged; an air of impatience proliferated alongside a booming technological world; and an accident left my father physically disabled and unable to speak, though with his wits intact. The typewriter became a dinosaur, too cumbersome and halting for the new era. The requisite pauses—to insert a new sheet, to align edges and margins, to return the carriage at the end of each line, to replace a ribbon with faded ink—were precious moments purloined by progress.

I could no longer think of my father as a purveyor of the written word. The typewriters he once fixed were now relegated to top shelves, attics and flea market stalls. And, with patience essential, my father would now point tremulously at a letter board to make his own words known.

Over time, my early love of writing re-emerged. But I wrote stealthily. I filled journal after journal and never showed a soul. I am always writing in my head; words tumble into my mind, already alive.

Sometimes words float up while I am running—the rhythm of my feet stir thoughts to line the meandering paths in my head, to give shape to an idea as yet unformed. One morning, a few months back, running along the canal, I felt particularly free and open. As mist rose above the water and tangled with branches hanging low over the canal, I caught sight of a great blue heron fluffing its wings, curling its beak below its outstretched feathers, with one beady eye fixed on me, unblinking. In that moment, words leaped into my mind, as though I was hearing them read aloud, as clear as the nearby warbler trilling in the thicket.

I stopped; I took out my phone and recorded my words, words arisen out of the mist.

#

Recently, I've been cleaning out my parents' New York City apartment, the apartment where I was born and where my parents lived for over six decades. It has been a strange and sideways journey. I am not efficient; I can't seem to throw anything away. I am my mother's daughter. Every object I hold sparks a memory, a scent, an image that returns me to my child self. I silently slide open the drawers in my mother's dresser, sniff her perfumes, run my fingers over her delicate powder-puff (now crusted over and tattered), open each tiny jewel-box and peer at the glittering stones tucked into their white cotton beds.

Cleaning out the top shelf of my mother's closet, I reach, and way to the back, where I cannot see what my fingers grasp, my hand closes around a dusty shopping bag, which tears at the seam as I pull it down. Inside, I find hundreds of letters written on old-style, extra-light, blue airmail letters. I open them up. Letters between my parents, during the year before their marriage, when they lived in separate cities, my father traveling weekly to visit. Pulling out a letter at random, I read my father's familiar scrawl:

> I cannot wait till I see your shocked face at the airport—you were not expecting me! And now I wonder, should I have kept my visit a surprise? Or should I have told you, so you could be as excited as I am right now waiting to see you? I'm looking out the window—we're in the clouds right now!

These words—written by a young man who was liberated less than a decade earlier from the Mauthausen concentration camp, who did not speak a word of English when he arrived in the United States five years later—take my breath away. I am transported to the cabin of that plane, where my besotted father adds to his letter every twenty minutes, nearly unable to contain the exquisite pleasure at this anticipated reunion. This stack of letters contains the hopes, the dreams, the agonies and traumas of a young man mourning a lost world at the same time that he reclaimed his life through the power of words. As I read each letter, I realize the importance of creating words, stories and narrative worlds in a home haunted by unspeakable losses, by ghosts of people I will never know and events I will never fully understand. Words lend form to the shadows of the past.

And suddenly I understand: this is why I write, why I've continued to write long past relinquishing my longed-for writer's life. Writing is an act of love, of memory, of desire, of restitution, of repair. Writing is a way to reclaim myself.

As I write this, images of my parents' early lives arise and shift around me. Their presence lingers beside me, peering over my shoulder, waiting to see what I have written, whether I succeed in breathing life back through the words on the page.

Carefully, I fold the letters, bind them together and carry them out of the apartment. I walk through the rooms one last time. The air is still. The ghostly presence slips away. Perhaps to rest, their story told at last.

Ha Jin

Writer, Professor

Writing as Salvation

One evening in the summer of 1988, Frank Bidart and I were having dinner at a Thai restaurant in Newton Center, Massachusetts. He was the poet-in-residence at Brandeis, where I was a third-year graduate student. I had just shown him my poetry manuscript, which later became my book *Between Silences*. He was excited about the poems, and we had been working on them. Over dinner we talked about poetry writing. He said, "Look, I'm almost fifty, but the best of me hasn't come out yet. I'm sure I will write better poetry." I didn't know how to respond to that, because back in China most modern and contemporary poets had reached their peaks before middle age. Frank's later poetic development has verified his claim—indeed he has produced more significant work afterward.

On the same occasion he also said, "If I hadn't written poetry, I would've been dead long ago." Again, I had no idea how to take that. At the time it sounded to me more like an expression of a personal sentiment. I did not understand what he meant, and again bit my tongue.

I was a beginning writer and had a great deal of misgivings about writing and about my future, which I envisioned as teaching American literature at a Chinese university while translating some literary books from English. But intuitively I felt that prospect might change. I was unsure whether I'd be able to come out of China for academic exchanges once I went back. I had seen that a whole generation of Chinese scholars and scientists educated in the States had wasted their lives, isolated and fossilized in China, so I feared I might repeat their lives despite my resolve to return. Later, the Tiananmen tragedy took place and I couldn't go back to China anymore. But I never stopped writing, because it was something I could do. Deep down I had some kind of hunger that only writing could satisfy, yet the act of writing was

DOI: 10.4324/9781003516118-38

no more than a way to spend my life. I didn't know what else I could do to alleviate the deep hunger.

This hunger made me respond to Kafka's "Hunger Artist" with intense poignancy. The nameless artist in the story fasts because he can't find any food he can eat. As a result, fasting becomes his way of existence and also his art. There is no celebration of this art, the performance of which actually originates from his sickness. Eventually, even the breaking of the fasting record doesn't mean anything to him anymore. Therefore, I couldn't see anything extraordinary or glorious in such a performance, though I understood the hunger and could commiserate with the hunger artist. For me, writing was a performance of that kind, morbid and solitary, since I couldn't do other things.

My understanding of writing was expanded by reading Chekhov. In March 1886, Chekhov received a letter from Dmitry Grigorovich, an elder novelist, out of the blue. In the letter the older man urges Chekhov to cherish his talent, stop writing tiny pieces for newspapers and undertake more serious literary work. He is convinced that Chekhov would be at the very front of his generation of Russian writers, so Chekhov must concentrate and quit working under the pressure of deadlines. Toward the end of the letter, Grigorovich says, "I do not know what your financial situation is. If it is poor, it would be better for you to starve, as we did in our day." The twenty-six-year-old Chekhov was moved almost to tears, and in his reply, told Grigorovich that he had scores of literary friends in Moscow, none of whom would bother to read his stories. Some even urged him "not to exchange the real business for scribbling." Chekhov was already a physician then; that must be "the real business" his friends referred to. He went on in the reply, "If I were to . . . read to them a single passage of your letter, they would laugh in my face."

Chekhov promised Grigorovich that he would work with more patience and a greater ambition. He said he wasn't afraid of hunger, "ready to starve," since he had gone through starvation before, but at the moment he couldn't do that yet, because he had family members to support. This is typical of Chekhov—humanity always comes first for him. Nonetheless, the great period of Chekhov began a few years later, during which he produced those glorious longer stories (the small masterpieces) and the magnificent plays.

The exchange between Grigorovich and Chekhov enlightened me and made me see the connection between writing and hunger, as if hunger was integral to literary creation. But then I realized that in the United States, hunger couldn't be an actual problem for a writer. As long as one worked some and was in decent health, one would not starve. I could work and wouldn't become a starving artist, even with a family to support. Materially speaking, writers in our time and in America are in a better situation than in the time of Chekhov and Kafka, when writers might have ended up starving physically for their art. This realization helped mitigate my guilt if I spent too much time writing, since I was certain that my family wouldn't starve as long as I kept a job.

Nevertheless, I didn't feel comfortable about the notion of writing as art. This was due to the fact that I had grown up in the revolutionary period of contemporary China, where pragmatism—the daily struggle for survival—had possessed people both physically and mentally. Art must be something useful, at least serving the people and society, and often also as a way of self-advancement. For a long time I wouldn't use words like "art" and "artists." During my eight years of teaching poetry writing at Emory University, I never used those words, and instead, would call a writer a "poet" or "fiction writer" and their art "work" or "poetry" or "fiction." Indeed, I never stopped writing, but it felt more like a physical need, and there seemed no metaphysical dimension to speak of. It was just something with which I could while away my life.

Yet about a decade ago, I began to use words like "art" and "artist." In some interviews given in Chinese, I surprised myself by claiming that I was an artist, not just a writer who produced books. Even though I noticed the change in myself, I couldn't clarify the reason for the change. Not until I realized there was some spiritual dimension in writing which I hadn't deliberated before. I noticed that among Chinese exiles and immigrants in North America, many had converted to Christianity or Buddhism. I admired them for their act of religious fulfillment, but I never felt the need. I often wondered why.

The major cause of anxiety and trauma among immigrants and exiles is the damage to their internal reference frames. This frame is a kind of mental grid, whose components include values, culture, religion, language, community, etc. Transplanted to a new land, one's internal reference frame is automatically altered or damaged or at times destroyed. As a result, one is disoriented and stressed. In some extreme cases, suicidal. This kind of damage is the source of fear and despair. Many Chinese immigrants and exiles who grew up in mainland China were ingrained with the values advocated by the communist regime. In that country, religions have been banned and mostly wiped out, so the only dominant values are rooted in materialism and patriotism. As a consequence, people, still possessed by religious longings, tend to deify the country. Worse, they can hardly differentiate the country from the state (the Chinese language has the same word for both, guojia, which further confuses the two in people's minds).

Therefore, the country has become God. Due to the linguistic confusion of the country and the state, many people simply identify the country with the ruling power, which is the party that controls the state. They equalize the party with the country, which must be absolute and sacred so that their religious longings can be satisfied. Most people back in China have ignored the fact that a country is a secular construct and often makes mistakes. Once the exiles and immigrants have landed elsewhere, their love for their native country can no longer sustain them mentally and spiritually, and the indoctrinated values cannot apply anymore. The very act of their departure already constitutes a kind of betrayal to their native land, so they have to seek another value system to repair their damaged internal reference frames, replacing the old obsolete values with new ones. Therefore, many of them have found that religion is a vaster system with a longer history, which can provide more universal and permanent values. In brief, religion can easily trump communism and nationalism. This explains why so many immigrants and exiles have embraced religion passionately. Indeed, religion—Christianity or Buddhism or Islam—can make them more steadfast in confronting the powers that be back in their native land. Religion helps them occupy a higher and firmer moral ground.

With my understanding of their psychological needs for religious conversion, I was still amazed that I had never been eager to do that, even though I have of course had religious longings. I often wondered: why am I different from those exiles and immigrants who have embraced a religion? Why wouldn't I join a church or a temple or a Koran class? Gradually, I figured out the reason—I have been writing and have gradually built a new value system in my internal reference frame, namely literature or literary art. In literature I have found a landscape or galaxy that is vaster and more enduring than a country or a state. In the literary constellation there are stars that can easily outshine most politicians and historical figures. Such a space is also divine and infinite, similar to a religion in its scope and depth. Therefore, writing has kept me steady, physically, mentally and spiritually. Fortunately, I have by chance entered the space of literature where I can find my own bearings. That explains why I am not that eager to adopt a religion. I can devote myself to the pursuit of the literary art, which can also transcend the constraints of patriotism and ideologies. In other words, I have been writing not only to satisfy the hunger within but also to help sustain my sanity and make my existence meaningful. This is the spiritual and existential dimension I was unaware of at the beginning of my writing practice.

After more than three decades, I finally came to understand why Frank Bidart claimed that had he not been writing poetry, he would have died long ago. He was speaking of the existential underpinnings he needed as an artist. That is also what I have needed. But not until lately have I realized that writing is also my salvation.

Kerry Malawista

Psychoanalyst, Writer

Why I Write: From the Faraway Nearby

On weekend mornings, my dad would open the door of his big red truck. He'd boost me up to the black vinyl seat, bow, and say, "Your chariot awaits you, Mademoiselle." What a treat to spend the day that way, just Dad and me.

Off we'd drive to a nearby New Jersey neighborhood, where we'd stroll down various streets putting flyers in mailboxes, "Leddy Siding" brightly festooned across them. Back in the truck, we would sing along with the radio and sleuth out the villain in the latest Nancy Drew series. When I ran out of books to chat about, Dad would ask, "Did you have any good dreams last night?" Dreams, he told me, held hidden clues. Together we cracked the code of those nighttime visions. To this day, I can't imagine how this man, who didn't go to college and never read a book (as far as I could tell), understood the importance of dreams and took mine seriously.

One Saturday, as "Bridge over Troubled Water" played on the radio, I was gripped by the lyrics. My mother was still alive then, so I know that I wasn't yet nine years old. It took my breath away to discover that "bridge" could mean a friend who helps you get over hard times. In that moment, I realized that words, like dreams, could hold multiple meanings. Words were the link between what lived inside me—thoughts, fantasies, memories—and the outside me, and I could use my words to connect myself to others.

This fascination with language's potential ignited my love of reading, and likely my desire to become a psychoanalyst.

What about my urgency to put words on the page? That came much later, sparked once again by the notion of a bridge. It was a year after my daughter died, when I still imagined catching a glimpse of her just around the corner or her coming home so I could tell her how unhappy I had been since she died. My husband and I were attending a Georgia O'Keeffe show at the Phillips Museum in Washington, D.C. Roaming the

DOI: 10.4324/9781003516118-39

galleries, I was taken with O'Keeffe's flowers of red, yellow and purple, each appearing as if under a microscope. But one painting in particular gave me an unsettled, off-kilter feeling.

The canvas showed the remains of a massive elk's skull and antlers suspended over a range of light-filled crimson mountains, rising up from the desert sand. I was struck by the juxtaposition: a bright, radiant light, and this looming marker of death. The title was printed in black letters on a white card at the lower left of the frame: "From the Faraway, Nearby."

Gazing at O'Keeffe's painting, I noticed the canvas lacked a middle distance. Without a middle distance the elk's bones—the marker of death—dominated the foreground, while the mountains were eerily distant. O'Keeffe had left out the bridge between them, their shared middle ground.

And with that title, I had words for how I had felt since Sarah's death. Sarah was still with me, unbearably yet thrillingly close, as though she might show up for the vegan dinner I'd cooked with her in mind. Living in my state of suspended disbelief, I could neither bring her back nor let her go. If I accepted she was gone, I feared Sarah would be lost to me—like being stranded off in the distance, in a mist settling over a distant mountain range.

O'Keeffe's painting and her four simple words, "From the Faraway, Nearby," gave meaning to what I was experiencing. Finding the middle distance was essential, a space to bear the unbearable and acknowledge the unreachable. I needed a bridge between the immediate and unending pain of losing my daughter and the desolate horizon of life without her.

Never thinking myself a writer, I jotted down thoughts first about O'Keeffe and then images and memories of Sarah. I was inscribing Sarah, and it allowed her to come to life on the page. Writing enabled me to reflect on the "before and after," create a narrative of what happened, and find words to both describe and ease my grief. Through this process, I built a bridge from the inchoate and disjointed memories to a bearable future.

Since then, embedded in all that I compose, whether a clinical chapter, essay, op-ed or novel, are themes of love, loss and connection. Each piece begins with the glimmer of a powerful moment, be it sad, joyful, humorous or confusing. I first share it vocally, honing my thoughts in conversation with an interested listener, and if the idea lingers and deepens, I take pen to paper. Initially there is no editing, revising or obsessing over language. My first aim is to get the words down, knowing that if I sweat the details I'll lose the essence of the story. When it's time for the task of revision, I dive into what I have penned, and new meaning comes to life. I revel in the magic of discovery, moving from the unknown to the known.

Psychotherapy is much the same pursuit, putting into words something imagined, felt or experienced by a patient. We explore not only what lies beneath and within those words but also the power they have over us. Together, writing and psychoanalysis offer me the opportunity to process experiences that exceed my initial understanding.

Writing opens me to self-discovery, and burrowing into the particulars of my own life reveals the paradox that personal truths are universal. As I rework sentences—over and over—connections spark, and the piece catches fire. I feel that I've succeeded when I hit an emotional beat that resonates with another, whether reader or patient.

Although loss, both my daughter and mother, first moved me to write, my work is suffused with all the joy my dad helped me discover. Jotting down those notes about driving with my dad transports me to those Saturday mornings of my childhood, cruising along in his work truck, supplies bumping and bouncing around in the back. Memories spring back to life: Dad's familiar smell of Brylcreem fills the air, as does the jaunty way he hummed along to the music. A pencil rested atop the earpiece of his Clark Kent glasses, with their smudged lenses, and as he drove, he'd squeeze my hand three times—a hidden message (I-love-you) and ask, "Did you get the message?"

Writing is my way of showing that I get the message.

Judy L. Kantrowitz

Psychoanalyst, Writer

" . . . or music heard so deeply
That it is not heard at all, but you are the music
While the music lasts."
—T. S. Eliot, from "The Dry Salvages," 1941

I no longer know when I first read these words, but I've never forgotten
them. They resonate with some inchoate experience of my own, something ineffable.

I am an only child. While I had a lot of friends, books always transported me to a special place; different, magical.

When I was five years old, I had typhoid. For months I was in bed, but
I remember only my mother reading me the entire *Wizard of Oz* series.
I loved it and delighted in the books again as I read them to my own children. Later, I read the whole Nancy Drew mystery series. A childhood
friend, still a good friend today, reminds me how we played at being girl
detectives. I made weekly trips to the Brooklyn public library, planning
to read straight through the As and Bs all the way to Z in the children's
section. Of course, I failed. Actually, it took me a long time to learn to
read. Maybe I wanted to continue to be read to? But books remained my
companions.

My school was a progressive one with an almost perverse investment
in making children feel good even when they weren't good at learning.
In 5th grade I purposely misspelled "bridge" to get that re-assuring attention. Little did I realize that I didn't need to try—to this day I am a terrible
speller, grateful to computers for spell check.

At age twelve, when I finished *Gone with the Wind*, I came sobbing
to my mother. She, who was usually empathic, said, "It's only a book."
Only a book! How could she say that? Long before I could read or go
to the library by myself, she had taken me there. She talked to me as
if I were an adult, confiding her childhood hurts, her current life disappointments. Her failure to empathize with my vicarious sorrow for

DOI: 10.4324/9781003516118-40

Scarlett bewildered me, stung me. Likely it was then that I began to separate from her. Even though I'm sure I didn't realize it at the time, that failure also primed me for knowing I wanted to go places she would not go, and would even discourage me from going. For I was on a trajectory, seeking emotional intensity, almost all still vicarious. And I found it in books.

So, no surprise: I adored Dostoevsky. All the tumult, the questioning. Faulkner was also compelling but too traumatizing. My own world seemed so cloistered, protected. My closest friend shared a love of music and art. We'd spend Sunday afternoons singing folk songs in Washington Square and wander for hours in the Museum of Modern Art. My mother was an artist but far too didactic a companion at that time.

My friend and I also shared our adolescent angst. And, like most teenage girls, I kept a diary—totally embarrassing to re-read now—filled with badly written, over-the-top emotions; there are only a few rare moments where I pause for reflection: "Sometimes after what you thought was a meaningful relationship ends, even if the feeling about the person fades, something associated with one's intense affect remains meaningful." I still love the song "Greensleeves," connected with a youthful crush. Music again. On re-reading the diary, I see how pleased I was by my own precocity.

In high school, I wrote some for the school literary magazine. As a freshman, I wrote a short piece that was published. Called "The Glass Wall," it was about wanting connection that could be perceived but not realized. A senior wrote in my yearbook how moved she had been reading it, and I was moved by her recognition.

Then came a story about a time I had surreptitiously taken some beads (even now I don't like to call it stealing) from a friend. A childhood experience of guilt and reparation transformed in this tale. Years later, when interviewed for admission to psychoanalytic training, the interviewer asked me what I had wanted to be when I was a child. When I said, "a writer," he asked me to associate to something I had written. The stolen bead story came to me. I was flooded with old feelings and regressed in a fog of memory, desire, guilt. I left the interview in a fog, trying to recover and reconsider what I had said and learned about myself.

Beads that could become a necklace . . . maternal, feminine, gorgeous. Yes, I had wanted them, but the wish had been forbidden; until then, unknowable. Could I have asked for them? Could I allow myself to find my voice? No, I had to steal. My mother told me her mother told her that for a woman to work was to be a prostitute. Could I defy this proclamation? Was it greedy to want it all: to be a wife, a mother—a writer?

I had thought I wanted to be a writer. I wrote one, maybe two, credible short stories. In college I suffered through a brief unrequited love, and then as a sophomore met my husband. We fell in love quickly, decided to marry. To join him geographically while he finished his professional training, I transferred to Sarah Lawrence. My imaginative arc suffered as my happiness soared. The passion for reading, however, was greater than ever. Sarah Lawrence was an intellectual paradise—small seminars, one-on-one tutorials with scholars like Joseph Campbell. Intellectually, I was happier than I ever could have imagined.

But what was I going to do in my own professional life? I knew by then I didn't have the talent to be a fiction writer, and I didn't want to be an academic: as much as I loved literature, the strictures of an academic classroom, the pressures to publish all seemed confining. I wanted more freedom. I presented my quandary to Gerard Fountain, the school psychiatrist, a psychoanalyst who had been an editor of the *Psychoanalytic Quarterly*. Fountain was known for his passion for literature. He asked me what I loved. I answered, "Literature, character development." "Not science?" "No, not science." He said, "Go to social work school." I didn't follow Gerard Fountain's advice exactly, but our conversation led to my deciding I wanted to be a clinician.

For the next ten years, I wrote to meet academic requirements: papers, a dissertation, a piece of research. Then, for almost twenty years I wrote to persuade, to argue for a conception of psychoanalysis in opposition to the dry ego psychology many were taught in the late 1960s. And yet, my writing was also gradually becoming less theoretical, or abstract, and more personal. Over time, I had begun to write about my work with patients: how we affected each other, what I learned from them, not only about them but about me. I could observe a process between us that broke down when something in myself kept me from listening well-enough, when my emotions, or their resistance, was more than I could bear. I wrote about how I'd fail to recover, and sometimes did recover, but other times not sufficiently. I was in the process of discovering the effect of what I termed the psychoanalytic "match" between patient and analyst, a factor that could "enable or disable" the process. I loved this writing about character and conflict. I was telling how it happened, what evolved, what didn't happen, evoking the pleasure and the pain: how and why we reached an impasse, how we resolved it, if we could. It was like a mystery story, something hidden, but there were clues the patient and I could put together in the process of discovery. Reading had helped me know myself and now writing did the same.

Writing and publishing about the match also brought me new friends. I exchanged letters with others who were seeking to broaden the profession's perspective. Some of these friendships became deep and lifelong, an intimacy found through shared work. Although an only child, I no longer felt alone. My family through friendship became larger, and I was part of an even larger world of people I didn't know who shared my outlook on life and my passions.

And always, alongside my work with patients, I read novels. Always, the vicarious pleasure of entering others' worlds and minds—through my patients, as they conveyed their struggles, and through books in which authors brought characters alive with their understanding and gift with words.

And I wrote.

But what was I doing when I invited a large number of analysts and then later former patients to tell me about their experiences? In one project, I invited authors from around the world to discuss their choices in protecting the confidentiality of patients whose stories they published. What were the ramifications of these decisions, for the patients, for our fund of knowledge? Though I am interested in ethical dilemmas, this was not my usual kind of topic. And why did I invite former patients to talk about the ending of their treatments, their terminations? Ostensibly, I had chosen topics that were controversial, challenging a theory that to me seemed outmoded and limiting. I believed that now we knew more, and certainly we no longer accepted that one suit fits everyone. Although both were fields of valid enquiry, why did *I* take these topics on?

A colleague-friend asked me this very question, noting how different this writing was from most of my other writing. I responded without thought: I was working like a reporter. And then, I felt an inner churning: five years earlier our thirty-one-year-old son had died of a brain tumor; he had been a reporter. By entering his world, was I keeping him with me?

Ten years later, I presented a paper about the analyst, enabled and disabled by what is personal; and my colleague-discussant wondered: had the loss of our son also led me to work on the issue of termination? The answer was: Yes. Of course. But each time, I had not made the connection until my colleagues, both women, brought it to my attention. By not knowing the link to my grief, was I protecting a privacy that had been hard to preserve in childhood? Was the pleasure I allowed myself at this discovery increased because the understanding came from two female colleagues? Their insights felt like gifts, not intrusions. And I had to wonder: did my writing also reflect the work to separate from my mother, keeping her with me as I found my own voice all along?

I recall still another project. In the mid-1990s, I invited psychoanalysts in the United States to answer questions about how their patients had affected them. To all appearances, I was continuing my interest in the patient-analyst match and seeking to make countertransference responses a normal part of the relationship (it's hard to believe this was still a needed contribution to the field, but it was). Most of the analysts who responded were male, "confessing and confiding," as one of them put it, experiences in which they felt ashamed of their responses to their patients. As I listened, I thought of my father who had not been able to tell me the story of his father, a gambler, who had deserted the family when my father was six years old. Yet repeatedly he came home, impregnated my grandmother, took the money she made managing a dry goods store and left again. Until my father's older brother, then twelve, said, "Enough! This time we are locking him out." And they did. As my mother eventually confided in me, my father and his brother helped their mother raise the three younger children while attending school and earning money making deliveries for the dry goods store. To me, there was nothing shameful in this story. But my father saw it differently. He did not want me to know. Until my father's death, I believed his father had died of a heart attack when my father was six. My father's two younger brothers had died of heart attacks in their forties and my father expected an early death would be his fate. He actually died at the age of seventy-eight in 1980. As I listened to the confessions of these older men, I knew I wanted to help them with their shame in a way it was too late to help my father.

But I realize only now that my unconscious motivation as I wrote was to mourn my father, to keep him alive in my mind. My father had died toward the end of my analytic training, fifteen years earlier. Everyone loved him—he was warm, giving, funny, fun. I miss him still, like I miss my son. I now grasp that all three of the books in which I interviewed others were my way of grieving. But my grief had not reached the layers where I was keeping lost and beloved members of my family with me, despite consciously accepting their absence. Perhaps grieving in this fashion preserved a privacy often hard won in my childhood. I think of Tony Kris, who wisely corrected Freud's idea about mourning. We must indeed mourn and relinquish our hope for a future with a beloved person who dies, but we need never lose the past. What we shared is ours to keep.

I still wish I had that fiction writers' gift to transform what is personal into compelling stories. For me, though, writing may satisfy a hidden wish to be a detective, to discover something previously unknown in myself, something that may subtly change me. Perhaps I have found a link between being a psychoanalyst, a writer and a reader. I continue to immerse myself in novels, especially those in which characters evolve and relationships deepen, with language that is beautiful, heartful and evocative. Reading connects me to that place Eliot describes, to a music that is deeper and broader than the words themselves. I learned what I didn't know I knew, but needed.

David Litt

Speechwriter, Author

The Reader Makes it Real

In 2007, at the start of my senior year of college, I went to brainyquote. com, copied and pasted a few selections, printed them out on colored paper and covered the walls of my room with the laminated results. I hoped they would inspire me. More than that, I hoped they would inspire women to have sex with me.

For obvious reasons, it didn't work. Even at twenty-one years old, I must have realized no potential romantic partner would cross my threshold, see the Will Rogers quote *Even if you're on the right track, you'll get run over if you just sit there,* and rip her clothes off.

So why did I do it? What did I really hope to achieve?

Maybe I just loved words. The way Rogers—or Twain, Ephron, Parker and the rest of my wallpaper canon—could take the nucleotides of language and organize them into something pulsing and alive. Perhaps I felt called to one day be like them, to stand on their shoulders as best I could, to be (insert long, dramatic pause) . . . a writer!

What a noble person I would be if any of that were true. But I didn't think of myself as a writer back then, aspiring or otherwise. A far better explanation of my senior year décor is captured nicely by a quote from the British novelist E.M. Forster, whose last name I spelled "Forester" on the laminated sheet taped above my dresser:

How do I know what I think until I see what I say?

Forster was born nearly a century before I was. Yet he captured something that, at twenty-one, I hadn't realized I was feeling: a deep certainty that there must be more to me than me. My self—the flawed vessel that frequently combed its hair with a fork and attended campus parties wearing an Indiana Jones hat, a thrift-store blazer and pajamas—contained something special, something elegant and powerful and meaningful and as-yet-unexpressed.

Before I could fall in love with writing, however, I discovered a different form of self-expression: politics. The night of the 2008 Iowa

DOI: 10.4324/9781003516118-41

caucuses, I watched a young senator named Barack Obama give a victory speech. "Faced with impossible odds, people who love this country can change it," he told the crowd. A wall-worthy quote if there ever was one. Yet Obama was nothing like the navel-gazing Forster. Before the speech was even over, I knew that I was about to embark not on a journey of self-discovery, but a something-bigger-than-myself-discovery. Politics might not be creative. But it could be expansive.

It never occurred to me that these distinctions might be artificial, that politics could be a means for self-expression or that writing could help people reach beyond themselves. Even stranger, my life had been changed forever by Obama's writing, yet I still never considered becoming a writer myself. I worked as a field organizer during the general election, and when I moved to Washington afterwards, I hoped to find a job in healthcare policy.

One night I was introduced to a friend of a friend who was throwing a thirtieth birthday party. When she told me she worked for a speech-writing firm, I politely feigned interest, but inwardly I recoiled. *Writing for other people? Turning thirty?* Both prospects seemed unimaginably disappointing.

Then I discovered that finding a job is hard, particularly if you're not qualified for the jobs to which you're applying and you're graduating from college in the middle of a once-in-a-century economic collapse. I happened to meet the partners at the firm my friend-of-friend had mentioned. They offered me an internship, which quickly turned full-time.

That's how I became a professional writer. Not out of passion for words, or a desire to express myself. I began speechwriting because it was the first time in my adult life that people who were very good at something seemed to think I could become very good at that thing, too. As a recent graduate, writing was nothing more or less than the path of least resistance. I thought I would do it for a few years, then return to Obama's re-election campaign as a field organizer in 2012. But my path had even less resistance than I anticipated. I wound up getting a job as a speechwriter in the White House, first for the senior staff and then for President Obama himself.

I enjoyed the perks of my new job: tickets to the President's box at the Kennedy Center, access to the underground bowling alley. I saw *Hot Tub Time Machine* on Air Force One. How many Americans can say that? But as eagerly as I embraced public service, I still didn't think of myself as a *writer*. Speechwriting, I intoned when asked, is far more craft than art. Words are just tools, a means to reach a political or policy end. There's a reason that, within policy circles, speechwriters are often referred to as "wordsmiths." It's a compliment. But it's the kind of compliment that's laced with insult. It distinguishes speechwriters from real writers, separating the talented from the merely skilled.

The more junior the speechwriter, the more wordsmith-y the job. When I began writing speeches for President Obama, my primary role was to cut-and-paste. The first time I sat in on an Oval Office speechwriting meeting, the chief speechwriter ran through the calendar, starting with the highest-stakes remarks. As POTUS thought through the most important speeches, he would dictate thoughts, arguments, sometimes sentences or parts of paragraphs. But when we finally got to my set of remarks—so forgotten by history that even I no longer remember what they were about—he looked puzzled.

"We have language on that, right?"

He was. We did. I loved my job, but the bulk of it was to reassemble parts of old speeches into slightly new ones. I imagine it was a bit like being a suburban architect. You can add flourishes, but all the houses end up looking fundamentally the same.

Barack Obama was a memoirist before he was a politician, our first real writer-president since Lincoln. But he never seemed concerned when his less-significant remarks were works of competence more than creativity. In fact, that was one of his great strengths. Among speechwriters, certain politicians are infamous tinkerers, the kinds of people who will run late to a meeting with world leaders because they couldn't decide between "must" and "need to" in a set of remarks only a few dozen constituents will ever hear. Among Obama wordsmiths, on the other hand, there was a story—perhaps apocryphal—about a speechwriter who watched as the president read over those prepared remarks. Finally, the leader of the free world looked up.

"Okay," he said, satisfied. "We don't need a home run every time. We can hit some doubles, too."

For most of my time at the White House, and particularly for the first few years of it, I was assigned mostly non-home-run speeches. But here's the thing: when President Obama stepped in front of a crowd and gave those speeches, they weren't doubles any more. Being a junior wordsmith forced me, in a way few other types of writing would have, to pay attention to the audience. I watched faces as they listened. I heard bursts of laughter and applause. For the first time, I saw that writing is a two-way street, that even when the language is recycled, the reader makes it new.

When a line resonated or a joke landed, when the president crescendoed sentence upon sentence, magic happened. It was the same magic I felt reading Will Rogers on brainyquote.com, or watching TV on the night of the Iowa Caucuses. A secret handshake was initiated by the speaker, and then somehow reciprocated by an audience of total strangers.

As any visitor to my senior-year bedroom knows well, Ian Frazier once wrote that *A woods with a bear in it is real to a man walking through it in a way a woods with no bear is not.* Watching President Obama turn doubles into home runs, I began to realize that the audience—be it reader, viewer or listener—was what made writing real for me.

It turned out my understanding of E.M. Forster's effect on me had been as misguided as my spelling of his name. What he said in his brainyquote—*How do I know what I think until I see what I say?*—was about self-expression. But the moment I read his words, he expressed not himself, but me. I've never met Forster, and given that he's been dead for more than half a century I'm not likely to. Yet we've shaken hands. Those handshakes are what mattered. The quotes, like the words in a political speech, were just a means to an end.

After I left the White House, I began writing under my own name—books, op-eds, scripts. Yet even now, I struggle to think of myself as a writer. Not long ago I checked in at a doctor's office. When the receptionist asked, "Are you David Litt the author?" I somehow heard it as "Are you named Arthur?" and told her no. You don't need to be a therapist to see that I'm ambivalent about my profession.

Maybe that's because I so closely associated "writing" with the see-what-I-say impulse I had at twenty-one, the embarrassing desire to navel-gaze, accompanied by the even more embarrassing certainty that my navel was so much more interesting than anyone else's.

Writing remains, and I suspect always will remain, an act of ego. But on good days, that's not all I do. Just as words in speeches are mere tools, for me writing itself is now a means rather than an end, and the end is connection. It's the chance to be part of that magical handshake, to express myself and someone else at the same time.

At least once a week, sometimes once a day, I fantasize about new paths of least resistance: founding a startup, getting an office job, going to law school. What keeps me writing is the same, perhaps misguided, impulse that, in hindsight, inspired me to tape laminated aphorism to my walls. I want to be reminded I'm not alone.

Is writing the only way to reach out across distance and time to find yourself in another person, and them in you? Probably not. But it works for me, and it has for a while, so I think I'll keep at it—keep learning from it, keep doing my best to fill the woods we walk through with the bears that make it real.

After all, it's like Will Rogers once said. *Even if you're on the right track, you'll get run over if you just sit there.*

Bill Griffith

Syndicated Cartoonist, Graphic Novelist

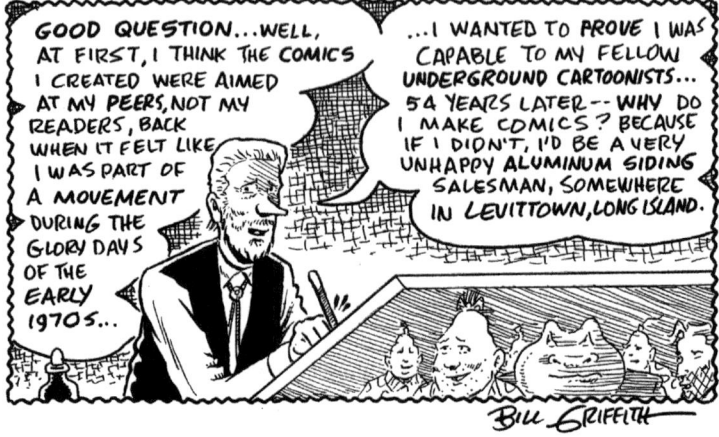

Figure 3.1

DOI: 10.4324/9781003516118-42

Peter Slevin

Reporter, Writer, Teacher

Why do I write? The first answer I can come up with: I don't know. I'd like to say something pithy: "I write because I must." Or existential: "If not writing, then what?" Or self-justifying: "If I don't inform the public, who will?" And maybe those are true, in a modest kind of way—but they weren't true at first.

At first, I just showed up for work. Not quite two weeks after I finished college, I parked my used Toyota Corolla, purchased a few days earlier with borrowed money, and took the stairs to the newsroom of the Hollywood, Florida *Sun-Tattler*, an afternoon daily in the Scripps-Howard chain. (Motto: *Give light and the people will find their own way*.) I had no greater purpose than to spend the summer gainfully employed, and no greater ambition than to conjure some ambition. Something happened, though, that gave me direction, purpose and ambition alike. I started covering stories. A two-year-old who fell into a backyard septic tank and died. A hurricane. A cop, goofing around in the squad room, who fired his gun and killed an innocent colleague. A Ku Klux Klan rally. A gubernatorial campaign. A police review board in a racially divided city. All of the life, and grief, that flowed through the local courthouse.

I can't pretend it was noble, but the work was exciting. It posed an intellectual and emotional challenge. It introduced me to unfamiliar worlds and taught me new things. On my best days, it felt useful. Just maybe, if I left the office and found the right voices and scenes, my stories would give someone an idea, or some perspective, or a laugh.

I have to emphasize the shakiness of the endeavor. Some stories were better than others. Daily journalism, with its demands and its deadlines, is no place for perfectionists. Nor did we usually know, at the *Sun-Tattler* or *The Miami Herald*, where I alighted after a couple of years, whether a story mattered or quickly disappeared. Back then, when stories were only delivered in newsprint, they didn't call it the fish wrapper for nothing.

But we had fun, and we cared. It was a privilege, then and now, to be paid to find things out and write them up. *The Herald*, in its freewheeling

DOI: 10.4324/9781003516118-43

heyday, was stacked with talented writers and memorable characters, all covering a city where truth was more fabulous than fiction, mainly because if it were fiction, no one would have believed it. Along the way, my own sense of purpose deepened. This was years before any of us felt the need to push back, hard, against the theatrical fakery of Donald Trump and the Republican allies who shouted "Fake News!" at the journalists who exposed their hypocrisy and misdeeds. We were not, as Trump would have it, enemies of the people. Quite the opposite, as we saw it. We were the people, showing up with pens and notepads, telling readers, however imperfectly, what was happening.

Locally, nationally, internationally, I burrowed into realms where so much needed to be exposed or explained, seeking out voices that were not always heard. The work started to feel like a responsibility—a worthwhile one. Plus, I felt a profound sense of obligation to my sources. So many trusted me with their stories or simply took time to educate me; how remarkable those people were. The more powerful the interviews and the more revelatory the reporting, the more I feared, as I started to type, that I would fail to do justice to what I had just heard and seen. In other words, that I would blow it.

I moved to Europe in the 1980s, when American newspapers were flush with money and ambition. Zelig never had it so good. As *The Herald*'s lone correspondent, I was free to roam. The troubles in Northern Ireland. The peripatetic Polish Pope. Live Aid. The first Gulf War. Glasnost, the Soviet coup and the stunning breakup of the Soviet Union. The triumph of Solidarity. The reburial of Imre Nagy. The protest marches in Leipzig. The fall of the Berlin Wall. The smooth Prague revolution and the messier one in Bucharest. The wonder of seeing two-cylinder Trabants putt-putting out of East Germany on their way to Paris. As rewards go, being on the scene was not just ample, it was extraordinary. How could I not feel a drive to describe, to explain, to witness—to write.

There was the summer morning in the Sistine Chapel when I climbed the scaffolding to talk with Piergiorgio Bonetti, an art restorer, who was cleaning centuries of candle smoke and grime from Michaelangelo's explosively colorful ceiling. That very day, he was tending to *The Creation of Adam*. I couldn't help but reach up and touch the outstretched hand of God. Who gets to do that?

Or the December afternoon in Leningrad, with the widow and son of Valery Sablin, the idealistic Soviet naval commander who led a doomed mutiny aboard the battleship Storozhevoy, the real-life drama that inspired The Hunt for Red October.

The surreal scene inside an Indiana prison, witnessing a federal execution that served no purpose but retribution. The hours listening to young Marines in Ohio describe their return from a jarring tour in Iraq. The days of despair in flooded New Orleans after Hurricane Katrina. The weeks in Cuba and Haiti, where too little ever changed.

And, of course, the unseasonably warm November night in Chicago, when one big thing did change, as Barack Obama became the next president of the United States.

An enduring conceit about being a correspondent is the image of the swashbuckler: the belted trench coat, the voice of authority, the nights of gallivanting. I found the opposite, nearly without exception, for the simple reason that such work, done well, is difficult. For anyone serious about getting the story, the effort is humbling, because you never know enough. That's why wags used to tell green reporters, parachuting into a country for the first time, "Write it before it gets complicated!"

At first, everything makes sense. Two days later, with a dozen more interviews in the notebook, nothing does. It's like the old story of the three correspondents sitting on a park bench in the Soviet Union, watching a dog chew on a stick. The one who just got off the plane says, "Wow, all dogs in Moscow are black." The second one, in Russia longer, shakes his head and says, "No, we only know that this dog is black." The group is silent for a minute, and then the third correspondent, an old-timer, says quietly, "Actually, we only know that this side of this dog is black."

Good writing depends on good reporting. A lyrical opening and a few turns of phrase can only take you so far. It's a happy synergy that my favorite thing, professionally, requires being out and about, talking with people and seeing for myself. When you start a story with questions, instead of answers, and you get out of the office and listen, you're going to learn things. As often as not, you'll be surprised, because the thing you thought you knew was wrong, or has changed, or has a facet that hadn't occurred to you. And then you get to tell people, in your own words, what you learned. What's better than that?

The final piece of the why-I-write puzzle is my pleasure in the puzzle of writing. It's the satisfaction of finding the right words and assembling the bits and pieces into a coherent whole. Or, as the editors in Miami used to say, making it sing. (More often than not, it only hums.) I learned that the hardest stories to report and write, the ones where I could spend an hour on a single paragraph and still not get it right, are the ones I remember longest and cherish most. A long time ago, I showed up for work in a small newsroom in an unfamiliar place and got to meet people and learn things and tell stories. I write for a bigger audience and a fancier publication now, but nothing, really, has changed. And that's a good thing.

Robert Jay Lifton

Psychiatrist, Author

On Being a Writer: My Story

We write because our sense of self requires us to write. But exactly what drives that requirement is never really clear. So we create stories about it.

My story begins with a walk in Hong Kong in late April of 1954, when I was twenty-eight years old. I wandered through the crowded colonial streets past small Chinese noodle stands and elegant European dress stores, but my mind was on neither the people nor the streets. I was painfully preoccupied with an important life decision I was trying to make.

I had been living in Hong Kong, together with my wife BJ, for about three months, staying in a garret hotel room that we somehow found comfortable. I had been interviewing both Westerners and Chinese who had been subjected on the mainland to a remarkable process called "thought reform" (or more loosely, "brainwashing"). The process was always coercive in its use of criticism, self-criticism and confession. But it also called forth powerful exhortation on behalf of a new Chinese dawn, seeking to bring about a change in identity from the Confucian filial son or daughter to the filial Communist (or Maoist), and to do so in hundreds of millions of people. With Westerners "reeducated" in prison, there could be considerable violence used to extract false confessions of secret espionage.

Hong Kong was supposed to be just a stop on a leisurely round-the-world trip that began in Japan, where I had arranged to be discharged from the military after two years of service as an Air Force psychiatrist.

I had joined the military only because of having been subjected to a "doctor draft," and sent to Japan and then to Taegu in Korea, though never close to a combat area. I found myself fascinated by East Asia and its extraordinary postwar directions.

My final military assignment was to interview repatriated American prisoners of war released from Chinese captivity in North Korea. The

DOI: 10.4324/9781003516118-44

interviews were done first in the South Korean port city of Incheon, just below the 38th parallel and the no man's land area dividing the two Koreas, and then on a troop ship called the General Pope on a fifteen-day-voyage from Incheon to San Francisco. The repatriated POWs had been subjected to an export version of thought reform, and the military environment imposed constraints on my encounters with them.

Mainland China was then mostly cut off from the Western world and in Hong Kong I met "China watchers"—scholars, diplomats and teachers, who were European, American and Chinese—with whom I had lively discussions about the appeal and excesses of the Communist revolution. They in turn were eager to hear my impressions, as a psychiatrist, of a thought-reform process they found confusing. They put me in touch with Chinese students and intellectuals, as well as Western missionaries and teachers, who agreed to be interviewed about the psychology of the process they had experienced. I was immersed in a powerful historical moment, experiencing both fascination and a sense of adventure.

But I also felt uneasy at being isolated from American institutions, from the serious business of psychiatric and psychoanalytic training and the proper pursuit of my professional career—that is, removed from the structures of real life. Besides, our money was running out.

I was very reluctant to leave Hong Kong but could not seem to imagine staying. BJ was game either way. Hence my solitary walk.

My conflict was played out by first making a "decision" that we could not stay in Hong Kong, and then within a day reversing that decision by submitting an application for a research grant that would enable us to do just that.

I would later comment that the military saved me from a conventional life and I have never shown it much gratitude. A friend of mine put things differently: "You did not make the decision, the decision made you." (Unsurprisingly, that friend is a Zen Buddhist.)

The decision made me a writer. Not consciously—the words writer and writing did not enter my conflicted inner dialogue. What did concern me was whether I could become a *psychiatrist in the world*, a vague but compelling image that contrasted favorably with one of spending most of my professional life in a comfortable New York therapy office.

In fact, I had already published a paper for the American Journal of Psychiatry about my interviews with returning prisoners of war. I was discovering, as others have, that no exploration of an event is complete—for others or oneself—until one writes about it, or at least puts it into some kind of mental structure.

In my case everything started with being a *listening writer*, with interviews that enabled me to take in the words of someone else as the basis for what I would write. Such listening came to anchor my work in general, whether with those Chinese or Westerners who had been "reeducated," Hiroshima survivors, Vietnam veterans or Nazi doctors. In those interviews I encouraged a back-and-forth that was much more of a dialogue than was any form of conventional psychiatric exchange. At the same time I kept what I called a "research diary," dictated immediately after the interview and making use of written notes I had made (mostly quotations from the interviewee). When I later organized my findings, I referred much more to this research diary than to the unwieldy tape recordings, though the latter were invaluable for checking on actual words expressed during the interview.

I was also, as I came to realize, a *witnessing writer*. I was aware of having unusual access to a process that was profound and troubling, and I wanted to retell it accurately and make it known, that is to bear witness to what I was learning.

My dictation did not stop with the research diary but extended to my overall presentation of my observations and interpretations. With thought reform and all other subsequent work, I have been a *talking writer*. Rather than the hand-brain interactions of most writers typing their work or even writing by hand, mine has been a brain-larynx connection. Even when I compose a blurb for a book or work on a short paragraph of any kind, I do so by speaking it into my Dictaphone, utilizing this old-fashioned instrument because it is more malleable than digital counterparts for quick shifts in spoken words. In all this, the computer screen (on which an assistant types my words) is of importance only to enable me to visualize what I have spoken in order to redictate subsequent drafts until I am satisfied with the words on the screen.

Friends have told me that this auditory method makes my writing more "conversational," which is true enough but there is more to it. Whether listening, or speaking, I almost instantly merge the auditory with the visual: what I heard from Hiroshima survivors enabled me to see immediately before me the terrible scenes of death and pain they described. It is possible that in some way my auditory emphasis gave special intensity to its visual translation.

This admittedly idiosyncratic method seems to feed my psychological and historical—that is, psychohistorical—imagination.

There is also an important factor of place and space. My sequence has been to obtain my verbal information out in "the field," whether that be Hong Kong or Hiroshima or Germany or some other country in Europe or Asia—though with Vietnam veterans the "field" was the United States.

I have then come "home" to my study, a place for me of isolation and reimagining, wherever that study may be. My "mother of all studies" has been a separate, renovated shack, with a glimpse of the ocean, adjoining my Wellfleet house, where I have been able to place thick folders of transcribed interview recordings and research diaries on solid oak tables to carry through my version of sorting and writing. But I have had smaller replicas of that study in other places, such as in New Haven, New York, or Cambridge, depending on which university I was affiliated with at the time. My study came to take on the character of a special space where, with considerable difficulty, I might find the words I need.

This is my story of becoming a writer.

Permissions Line: Excerpt from *Surviving Our Catastrophes*— Copyright © 2023 by Robert Jay Lifton. Reprinted by permission of The New Press. www.thenewpress.com

Robert Boyers

Editor, Writer, Professor

Towards and Against the "Merely Personal"

Most critics and essayists of my generation were taught that there was something unworthy, even trivial and embarrassing, in what was called "the merely personal." Those I admired didn't write about themselves, certainly not about their "feelings." The essays I loved by Susan Sontag were personal only in the sense that they were spoken in her distinctive voice and conveyed insights and judgments I came to associate with her. So, too, the essays of Lionel Trilling, Harold Rosenberg, Irving Howe and others who wrote for *Partisan Review* when I became a subscriber in 1962.

Though the New York intellectuals obviously had lives, and sentiments, and had thought a great deal about subjectivity and the unconscious, they tended not to reveal anything about their private lives. Not in their essays and cultural criticism. Trilling never spoke about his own fears, disappointments and neuroses in his great essays on Freud and neurosis. Sontag could well have spoken about her own sexuality when she was writing about *The Story of O* or Jean Genet or the culture of the 1960s, and yet she chose not to. When I became friends with older critics and thinkers like Sontag and Howe, I learned all sorts of things about them that inspired me to imagine how their work might have been radically different had they given themselves permission to open up about their secret lives, their unfulfilled desires and torments. But their books and essays were in the best sense—so I thought—impersonal. Never bland or timid, but also never confessional or confiding. If I hoped to do the kind of work I admired in such writers, I, too, would have to master that species of impersonality. So I believed.

My favorite teacher in elementary school was a man named Moe Klores, and on open school night in 1953 he told my proud parents how diligent a student I was, "and nice," while also noting that I was an unusually "good boy," maybe "too good." Why, he wondered, did I always—always—sit with my hands impeccably folded on the desk

DOI: 10.4324/9781003516118-45

before me? Did I seem to my parents somehow "worried," as if I feared somehow being found out? He was, he said, just a little "concerned," and hoped that I didn't think too much about breaking rules, doing something wrong. All of which my parents heard as an expression not really of concern but of affection and esteem. This man, they told me, thinks a lot about you. Thinks you're "too good." Isn't that strange? Maybe you shouldn't sit so straight in your chair, my mother suggested. Maybe play with your pencil a little when you're sitting there.

Though I became a political radical and a war resister during the period of the Vietnam war and occasionally got into trouble because of essays I wrote, I remained, in ever so many ways, a very good boy. The discipline exhibited by my elders in the New York intellectual community seemed to me a wholly worthy achievement, and I took it very much to heart, almost as if it had been not merely a summons but an imperative. The work I aspired to do as a critic and essayist was to be worthy of the example set by Sontag and Trilling and the others, and though both Irving Howe and Harold Rosenberg told me, on several occasions, to let my sentences breathe more than in my early writings, they never recommended that I exhibit my feelings or introduce elements of diaristic narrative.

Of course we now live in the time of the personal essay, which has infiltrated the practice of criticism and cultural commentary in several beneficial ways. Writers who would once have thought it permissible to write about themselves only in overtly memoiristic works will now often include anecdotage even in a book review. As Phillip Lopate notes, the essay form has opened up to "an infusion of raw honesty, vulnerability, and awkward admission."

Today, when I read the essays of Elizabeth Hardwick, one of the very great essayists of the mid-twentieth century, I find it extraordinary that she can write about the life and works of writers she admires without letting on that she did or did not share with them certain proclivities. When we sat together on a panel on "Liars & Lying" at the Guggenheim Museum in 1973, she wondered aloud why I didn't speak "more openly" about my own experience of the syndrome we were discussing, though her own remarks were not remotely confessional.

One of my favorite Hardwick essays, on "Boston," recently republished in Phillip Lopate's anthology on *The Golden Age of the American Essay*, contains no mention of Hardwick's tumultuous years with Robert Lowell in Boston's Beacon Hill. What but discipline, or mere convention, could have prevented her from sharing with her reader her own encounters with the "pretension," "respectability" and "unctuous" qualities she cites as characteristic features of Bostonians? Who were the "men of quiet and timid and tasteful opinion" of whom she speaks with hilarious and lethal disdain, and how did she get on with them when they met?

Did she dissemble and pretend to share sentiments she loathed? Did she not herself attend, when in Boston, what she calls, in her own quotation marks, the "nice little dinner party" for whom a proper Bostonian "would sell his soul"?

Though there is no trace of "objective neutrality" in Hardwick's essay, there is also not a trace of the "vulnerability" or "awkward admission" Lopate cites as characteristic features of the contemporary personal essay, and the honesty in Hardwick's relentlessly scathing portrayal is decidedly impersonal. When she writes, unforgettably, that "the detergent of bourgeois Boston cleans everything, effortlessly, completely," the judgment is from on high, allowing for no misgiving, no merely personal admixture of a contradictory experience. There is, so far as we can tell, no secret self to excavate, no scorching memories to mine as a presumable source for the pervasive animus that we find at once entertaining and provocative.

Of course there were models of the personal essay to admire and emulate long before it came to dominate the landscape. When I was young, I was shaken by the essays of James Baldwin and, in the two years (1965–1967) I taught high school in New York City, I introduced them to my students in spite of the fact that I was warned not to do so by our cautious, conservative school principal. Obviously Baldwin came out with things that were not only distressing but somewhat incendiary, and I wondered what my students would make of a sentence in which he says that he never met a Negro who did not hate Jews. Would I recommend to my students that they allow for an element of exaggeration in essays of this kind? Would I ever give myself permission to exaggerate in this way? Always impressive, I felt, was Baldwin's urgent interrogation of his feelings—"astonishment, curiosity, amusement and outrage"— his way of talking about himself while also placing his experience in a framework that made it somehow characteristic, symptomatic. Who else would be apt to write, "In so far as I reacted at all, I reacted by trying to be pleasant—it being a great part of the American Negro's education (long before he goes to school) that he must make people 'like' him." Would I ever feel comfortable ascribing to people like me—who came from a working-class, white, Jewish background—characteristic habits of thought?

What made it possible for Baldwin to get away with things that I would not think to get away with myself? Would I hope to own up to the very different kinds of "rage" and "contempt" that, according to Baldwin, "no black man can hope ever to be liberated from"? When I introduced Baldwin's essays to honors students at Flushing High School, I invited them to consider what allowed him to speak, simultaneously, for himself and for others somewhat like him. Could we, as writers, as thinkers, adopt such a stance? What might prevent us from so much as trying?

Funny, I suppose, that the kinds of questions I was raising with high school students in the Sixties stuck with me for another forty years, and that even now I'm not entirely convinced that I have answered them to my satisfaction. In some respects, my perplexity always had to do with my simple desire to write essays somewhat like those I admired; essays by writers who preferred not to venture into the naked self-interrogation I found in Baldwin, or in writers like the George Orwell of "Such, Such Were The Joys" and "Shooting An Elephant." I believed that I had a certain modest gift for the sort of thing I began to write and publish when I was in my early twenties, and the sense of self that formed as a result of my enlistment in the cultural conversations of the Sixties, Seventies and Eighties fueled my belief. I never fully got over my commitment to the rigorously probing and largely impersonal mode of argument I had come to write.

In fact it was good for me—so I felt—not to drive towards something else for which I had neither a burning desire nor sufficient confidence that I could bring it off. I seemed to myself someone whose proper work was defined by a long-established investment in the essay as an instrument wielded by public intellectuals, for whom the pursuit of truth and the exercise of judgment was an honorable and demanding enterprise. Stodgy, that sounds, even to me at this moment. But then I continue to love essays marked by the several virtues Phillip Lopate identifies as "skepticism . . . thinking against oneself, open ended speculation . . . avoidance of system, and refusal of dogmatism."

Odd, then, that I came to think about my own disposition in a new way only when I began, in my early fifties, to write and publish fiction. Like many academics I had begun to think of myself as a poet and fiction writer when I was in college and publishing in an undergraduate literary magazine. But that ambition came rapidly to an end when, only a year or two later, my first reviews and essays began to appear in *The New Republic, Partisan Review, Dissent* and other magazines, including my own quarterly, *Salmagundi*. So that's who I am, I decided. And, as I've suggested, there was ample evidence to confirm me in that conviction. About the stories I was writing in my fifties I didn't quite know what to think. When a small press publisher in New York brought out my one and only collection of short stories in 2005, and it rose and fell with astonishing rapidity, I could only wonder what might have been had I chosen the uncertain rather than the certain thing thirty years earlier.

And yet, and yet: there was something in the response to that book that stirred me in another way. There was an accent there, in the fiction, that was nowhere visible in anything I had published in hundreds of essays and a half dozen books. Call it a wildness, a barely controlled ferocity my friends had not heard in my essays. Something corrosive and disturbing. Something I didn't know I wanted. Not in my own writing. A nice boy. Maybe too nice. Hands neatly folded. Not much of that boy in the stories. And when I went out on the road to give public readings—more than twenty-five in a half year—I was shaken by the intensity of the questions put to me, many having to do with the sense that the stories were thinly disguised revelations of their author. A dangerous fellow, obviously.

So, turning again—as I knew I would—to writing essays, unable not to do the thing I did, I had the sense that something in me had changed. I wanted to get that accent of dangerous self-exposure, of the corrosive and disturbing, into the essays I would write. I wanted my way with dialogue to become a feature of the essays, to invent a way of introducing the spoken voice into the rhetoric of what would remain a vehicle of cultural observation and criticism. I would take pleasure still in constructing a coherent argument and in provoking dispute; would hope to provide illumination, but with a considerable emphasis on my own subjectivity. In what I would set out to write I would hope to convey the problematic status of truth-telling, in part by telling the stories I had it in me to tell—working to "liberate" them, as Denis Donoghue wrote, and thereby disclose a "hidden face."

More, of course to say, about what all of this entails, or might entail. But it is certain to say that the answer to "why we write" is likely to be obscure, even to those of us who believe we are in possession of an indisputable answer. W.H. Auden, borrowing from E.M. Forster, wrote that he didn't know what he thought until he saw what he said, and I imagine that is one way of assigning a motive to our writing. We wish to know what we think. But I prefer to say that we don't know who or what we are until we see what we say, and that when we tell stories about ourselves, and expose ourselves to our own unsparing scrutiny, we are on the way to something we can almost believe in. This is something not entirely congruent with the objectives public intellectuals and cultural critics assign to themselves, but I like to think that the virtues of one pursuit are compatible with the virtues of the other.

Misgivings, to be sure, about these so-called compatibilities and virtues. As I survey the terrain of the paragraphs I've just composed, I miss the prodigal vagrancy I like so much in younger essayists who don't feel at all obligated to cover a territory or scrupulously investigate an "out there" we are, all of us, condemned to live in. The personal I have learned to draw out of myself, the stories I have come to tell, are never *"merely* personal," never a raw expression of appetite or desire. They are always in service, harnessed to an argument or to the exposition of an idea or a set of cultural conditions. In fact, most of the personal essays I read seem to me deficient in the degree that they are merely personal.

I remain, in spite of what has happened to my sense of myself as an essayist, committed to an exercise that is decidedly purposeful. I can't banish or censor the part of myself that wants the essay to be more than a performance and more than an opportunity to create a creative frisson. I want to sound more or less like myself, to be true to the nice boy who continues to demand that I at least pretend to be doing the right thing; in this case, trying to get to the bottom of something that seems urgent. Lots of opportunity for delusion in this line of work. Truth-tellers are always at risk of denying what else is wanted when you tell yourself that you want only to be truthful, your stagings and devices only a means to a worthy and certifiable end.

Lloyd Schwartz

Poet, Critic, Teacher

I Didn't Want to Write

And then I didn't want to do anything else.

In high school, I didn't like writing—didn't like the books we had to read. *A Tale of Two Cities. Silas Marner.* They meant nothing to me. Later, I was intrigued by the questions on a statewide exam. The subject was comedy. We had to read Bergson and George Meredith and look at paintings by Paul Klee. I already had a comic (and sinister) Klee on my bedroom wall. But I didn't look forward to writing answers. I wanted to be an architect. Or an actor. Neither of which required writing.

But in my senior year, I had an English teacher—Allen Kanfer (I didn't know his first name at the time), who reminded me of Groucho Marx (why am I not surprised that his son later became Groucho's biographer?). He'd do anything to get us excited about poetry. I still picture him leaping onto his desk, holding out his empty hand and declaiming: "Is this a dagger that I see before me?" Mr. Kanfer convinced me that Keats's "Ode on a Grecian Urn" actually *meant* something, and so did Frost's "Fire and Ice." I suddenly wanted to write something that meant something too. I knew I could never write anything as beautiful as Keats. Or as ingenious as Frost. So I wrote something silly, something (as I think back) that deliberately undermined the predictability of rhyme or what "poetry" was supposed to be. It was supposed to be funny. It wasn't very good, but it was my own—my first version of what could be a poem.

I was now in love with words and books and I wanted to write more poems. I wrote "serious" poetry in college. I took a poetry workshop (my only one ever), though my teacher didn't seem especially interested in my poetic ambitions or in helping me find my own voice. But I *was* ambitious. I became poetry editor of the school literary magazine, appropriately and without irony called *Spectrum.*

DOI: 10.4324/9781003516118-46

In graduate school, academic work was brutal. But I managed to have some sort of love life and I *had* to write poems about that. I'm not sure I realized how much my own poems sounded like everyone else's.

One turning point was reading a poem by a classmate. I was impressed by its intellectual complexity, but I didn't like its rhetorical language. So I rewrote it, leaving out everything I thought bombastic or self-consciously poetic. The original was two pages long; my version was two short stanzas. I showed it to another poet friend, who agreed it was a considerable improvement. Of course, it wasn't my poem, though it seemed more mine than anything else I'd been writing.

Was it shyness that, when I wanted to write a poem about sex, I didn't want it to be a confessional poem? Then it occurred to me that if I had a subject, I didn't have to be autobiographical—the way an actor inhabits a character, maybe someone as different from myself as possible—in gender, age or physical attraction. There was, of course, a long history of "persona" poems, but this poem would be really new for me.

This breakthrough triggered more poems in the voices of a wide variety of other people, both real and imagined. And these character poems, which I felt both more encouraged by and increasingly compelled to write—to stop everything to write them—seemed more my own poems than anything autobiographical I'd ever written. The language wasn't beautiful, but I thought the sound of a voice speaking was.

And these poems had an urgency missing from my earlier poems. A friend wrote to me that these new poems seemed to keep asking: "What about these people? What about these people?" So I called my first book *These People*. (It still bothers me when someone misremembers that title as *Those People*, which was the opposite of what I thought my poems were about—the way we are each one of *us,* not one of *them.*) That book got one bewildering review in which the critic thought all the poems, in their multiplicity of voices, were about myself. But in some unintentional way that reviewer may have been right.

Soon, the poems dealing with my closest relationships, lovers and (even harder to write) friends, were, unlike my old confessions, becoming dialogues, conversations and using increasingly eccentric devices: poems that offered more than one side to the story.

Even more urgent were the poems I began to write about my mother. In her late 80s, she was clearly developing dementia. She had always been a remarkable woman. I like to think she was the first woman in Brooklyn to drive a car, to get a telephone and a radio. She had to drop out of school after junior high so she could take care of her parents. Though she was born in Russia, she was the youngest and most "American" of her family and became a surrogate mother to the children of her old-world siblings. She was nearly forty when she married. I was her first and only child.

My mother was generous, funny, loving and I adored her, like everyone else who knew her. Before I could read, she read to me. Then taught me to read. I think she could have been a great teacher. Instead, she was a bookkeeper for a shady garage opposite Yankee Stadium (which is why, even though we lived in Williamsburg, I was a passionate Yankee fan), but retired from work when she married my father.

During her dementia, she told stories about her childhood and made uncanny pronouncements I didn't want to forget. I began writing down whatever she said, utterances that seemed a kind of poetry. "You're an apple," she said to me, "I'm a tree." Transcribing her "poems" became a calling.

#

Increasingly, I was also feeling how necessary it was for me to teach, especially poetry and poetry writing. Not, I hoped, like my college teacher. My role model was Robert Lowell, not from any course I took with him but from the free-wheeling "office hours" he offered at Harvard. Like his friend Elizabeth Bishop, Lowell was driven to write, though Bishop fought harder against her urges to write poetry. It could take her as long as twenty years to finish a poem, though Lowell was at least as compulsive a reviser as Bishop. *Revise, revise, revise,* she wrote about Lowell in her elegy for him. He would say you could do anything in a poem if you placed it properly. And though both of them could ascend to the most sublime heights, they both had extraordinary gifts for making great poems out of the most demotic language.

In some way I was closer to the Bishop model than to the Lowell. When I was hit by an idea, I dared it to leave me alone. I tried to ignore it until I couldn't ignore it any longer. Nothing was more important to me than writing poems, but I would fight off the impulse to write until I couldn't anymore. If the impulse went away, the poem probably wasn't worth writing. But when it took over, everything else got shoved aside.

With the poems about my mother, there wasn't time to make excuses. I was seized by them—they had to get written. I just had to figure out how to place everything properly. The title poem of my book *Little Kisses* ends with my mother singing me an old song, as she did when I was a child. "Little Kisses" began as one section of a longer poem called "Grief." Even after that poem got published, the section about my mother kept nagging at me. I just hadn't said enough—that poem really hadn't been written. The section about my mother from the earlier poem finally became part of what is now its own poem.

My own work ethic was not a great role model for my poetry students. What right had I to demand from my students an orderly writing life when I never did? But of course they were taking my workshop because they wanted to write, and improve. I could teach them that there was a difference between craftsmanship, which they needed to learn, and writing what *had* to get written. I rarely gave "prompts." I wanted them to write the poems they needed to write, not just finish assignments. Experiments, especially with traditional forms, were of course useful. I was thrilled when their experiments turned into revelation, as what might happen in my own poems if I was lucky or truly inspired. And some resistance was often a good thing. "Too easy" was rarely helpful.

#

In graduate school, on a tight budget, I discovered that if I reviewed student performances for the undergraduate drama reviews, I could get free tickets. I also enjoyed the freedom of writing critical prose—surprisingly different from the term papers to which I was painfully resistant, although they must have helped prepare me for the prose writing that surprisingly became an essential part of my life.

Reviewing had never been a particular ambition, but I took to it immediately. I liked the *idea* of being a professional writer. And I liked seeing my byline in print, and my opinion—usually different from what the other critics were saying. My own voice was becoming part of a public conversation. Literally my own voice when I started reviewing for the radio. I also had serious, thoughtful editors. I was mostly describing music, then visual art, especially painting. I'm still in love with the challenge of trying to capture music and art in words—different from writing poetry, though not always radically different. It was in my prose, not my poems, that I discovered I had a gift for metaphor.

In my reviews, I disliked using—as I disliked reading—technical descriptions. I wanted them—as I wanted my poems—to "speak" to whoever read them. Just as I admire music and art that seems to speak to me. *Talk* to me.

Poetry is still more important to me than prose. When I won an award for criticism, I told an interviewer that I hoped the award would encourage more people to read my poems (which probably never happened). But the differences between the two, sometimes very subtle, overlap in the impulse to show the beauty of spoken rather than traditionally literary language—speaking to the reader in either a poem or a review is for me the most compelling kind of writing.

Lately I've become interested in—*obsessed with*—turning some of my reviews into poems, or writing poems that almost sound as if they were reviews. I know it's an oddball choice, but it's both challenging and satisfying to finally bring these two aspects of my writing life together. So if someone tells me my reviews are like poems, or that my poems sound like my reviews (perhaps neither intended as a compliment), that still gives me a special, secret pleasure.

Peggy Tighe

Lawyer, Mentor, Writer

Writing Succinctly, a Journey

> At the bottom of her heart, however, she was waiting for something to happen. Like shipwrecked sailors, she turned despairing eyes upon the solitude of her life, seeking afar off some white sail in the mists of the horizon. She did not know what this chance would be, what wind would bring it her, towards what shore it would drive her, if it would be a shallop or a three-decker, laden with anguish or full of bliss to the portholes. But each morning, as she awoke, she hoped it would come that day; she listened to every sound, sprang up with a start, wondered that it did not come; then at sunset, always more saddened, she longed for the morrow.
>
> —Gustave Flaubert, *Madame Bovary*, 1856

For Catholic school girls in the 1980s, our literature "choices" were dictated by nuns and priests seeking to properly shape a young mind. We read overly descriptive sentences with tortured analogies meant to uncover feelings of ennui or unrequited love, inner struggles for more fulfilling futures and the right and wrong paths toward morally guided maturity. Sometimes we read "current" social commentary—*Madame Bovary* or Nathaniel Hawthorne's *The Scarlet Letter* (both published in the 1850s). Flaubert's heroine, who we called "Madam Ovary," longed for romance and wealth, which made her swallow arsenic and die a painful death. Hester Prynne didn't fare much better. We secretly read *Are You There God? It's Me, Margaret*.

Our teachers told us that real writers write beautifully detailed emotional prose; the longer the sentences the better. College brought a new twist: removal of feelings, inner turmoil and dew drop gazing, but still tediously long sentences.

DOI: 10.4324/9781003516118-47

Those of us majoring in political science and planning a law career could now pattern our writing after great philosophers and political theorists, or so we thought.

> A state also of equality, wherein all the power and jurisdiction is reciprocal, no one having more than another, there being nothing more evident than that creatures of the same species and rank, promiscuously born to all the same advantages of Nature, and the use of the same faculties, should also be equal one amongst another, without subordination or subjection, unless the lord and master of them all should, by any manifest declaration of his will, set one above another, and confer on him, by an evident and clear appointment, an undoubted right to dominion and sovereignty.
> —John Locke, *Second Treatise of Civil Government,* 1689

Writing like a legal scholar, as Locke demonstrates, must mean replacing feelings with reason typified by repetition of one thought expressed with multiple clauses adding a slight nuance to the original thought with the adroit use of multiple forms of punctuation. Political science majors could write hundreds of words; we simply had to say the same thing sixteen different ways, and preferably in one sentence. Locke's defense: "The way it has been writ in, by Catches, and many long Intervals of Interruption, being apt to cause some Repetitions. But to confess the Truth, I am now too lazy, or too busy to make it shorter." If we only knew then that Locke was—by his own admission—too lazy or too busy to write succinctly.

English majors, or in my case English minors, didn't fare much better, as illustrated by Dickens:

> It was the best of times, it was the worst of times, it was the age of wisdom, it was the age of foolishness, it was the epoch of belief, it was the epoch of incredulity, it was the season of Light, it was the season of Darkness, it was the spring of hope, it was the winter of despair, we had everything before us, we had nothing before us, we were all going direct to Heaven, we were all going direct the other way—in short, the period was so far like the present period, that some of its noisiest authorities insisted on its being received, for good or for evil, in the superlative degree of comparison only.
> —Charles Dickens, *A Tale of Two Cities,* 1859

Yes, that's the entire quote. That's why most people stop the quote at "it was the worst of times" because it gets much worse and certainly much longer. Lucky English majors—that is, those who didn't change majors after slogging through Chaucer's *Canterbury Tales* and

Beowulf—discovered Shakespeare, Edgar Allen Poe and Mark Twain. We were treated to the joy and challenge of writing concisely, as explained in two often cited quotations.

> Therefore, since brevity is the soul of wit, And tediousness the limbs and outward flourishes, I will be brief.
>
> —William Shakespeare, *Hamlet,* 1609

> I didn't have the time to write a short letter, so I wrote a long one instead.
>
> —Attributed to Mark Twain but more likely Blaise Pascal, 1657

Shakespeare's "brevity is the soul of wit" is wonderfully ironic because the verbose Polonius utters it briefly before he is stabbed to death. Twain's quote, according to literary historians, is often attributed to him but is more likely an abbreviated thought stated hundreds of years before by several people, most notably John Locke—the lazy, busy guy.

Given such literary role models, the way forward for writers aspiring to be pithy was as clear as a Locke treatise written by Dickens translated into French by Flaubert. I was fortunate enough to stumble into journalism.

Eliminate the extraneous to get to the bleeping point. Genius. That's why news writing begins with a strong lead and the five Ws: Who, What, When, Where and Why. Get their attention, tell them the facts. How refreshing for exhausted liberal arts students getting smarter very slowly. Early journalism was tied to "old media technology" such as the teletype or the use of molten metal to print each letter of a news story. Cleveland, Ohio, this writer's hometown, was named after Connecticut surveyor Moses Cleaveland, spelled with two a's.

> The common explanation was that the Cleveland Advertiser dropped the letter because it wouldn't fit on the masthead for its first issue in 1831. Case Western Reserve University history professor John Grabowski says that might not be totally true either: 'In their first issue they printed a box saying, 'Our subscribers will notice we are spelling it without the second 'a' because we think it's superfluous,' says Grabowski.
>
> —Excerpt from *Cleveland Magazine* (2019)

Lesson learned; journalists solved practical puzzles of molten lead by deleting the superfluous, even duplicate letters in people's names. To Flaubert, Madame Bovary was bored and anxious. To Dickens, the era was contradictory, like today. To Locke, people are equal. To Shakespeare, be brief though I am not. To Twain, borrow fewer words than others used.

What next for a would-be writer? For me, law school, where I saw English prose disemboweled for sentimentality and journalism shunned as an unseemly technical pursuit. I didn't have time to fret given the volumes of cases to read. One of the most important cases in American law, establishing the principle of judicial review, is *Marbury versus Madison*. It contains all the wordiness, redundancy and passive voice of English prose devoid of emotion but for pedantic indignation.

> If it had been intended to leave it in the discretion of the legislature to apportion the judicial power between the supreme and inferior courts according to the will of that body, it would certainly have been useless to have proceeded further than to have defined the judicial power, and the tribunals in which it should be vested.
>
> —U.S. Supreme Court, *Marbury versus Madison*, 1803

Since the 1800s, legal educators have made significant advancements in succinct legal writing. It took them a while. Law students still must read this horribly written legal brilliance. It is a logical conclusion that thousands of sentences absorbed by the average law student must be responsible for the death of lawyer brain cells responsible for processing English grammar. Read a contract or a legal disclaimer and tell me I'm wrong.

The next step in my *Gulliver's Travels* journey of effective writing was to heed the advice of writer Kurt Vonnegut:

> Find a subject you care about and which you in your heart feel others should care about. It is this genuine caring, and not your games with language, which will be the most compelling and seductive element in your style. I am not urging you to write a novel, by the way— although I would not be sorry if you wrote one, provided you genuinely cared about something. A petition to the mayor about a pothole in front of your house or a love letter to the girl next door will do.
>
> —Kurt Vonnegut, *How to Write with Style*, 1985

Writing about things you care about led me and many other lawyers to write to inspire action. Lobbying. Or, as Vonnegut said, getting the mayor to fix the pothole. Getting action from the next-door neighbor is a very different pursuit. I use persuasive writing as a legislative strategist for transplant surgeons and patients, Ryan White Clinics and people living with HIV/AIDs, safety net healthcare providers, physicians and cancer patients. Success for those audiences means advancing, modifying or defeating legislation.

The beauty of legislative writing is that it takes many forms—legislation, witness testimony, questions by members of Congress to witnesses, floor speeches, press releases, quotes on issues/events, issue papers, talking points and alerts to advocates on key issues. The more succinctly stated the better. I write to enlist allies to internalize and repeat what my clients believe, which I then help translate into law and regulation. As a new lobbyist, I often heard my lawyer friends say, as if I had a dread disease—"So, you don't *practice* law." My response: "I make law."

This writer's journey is one of many misguided attempts to mimic authors of classic literature, political theorists, philosophers and journalists. That journey brought me to legislative advocacy—a place where feeling, thinking, reason and persuasion all live in peaceful coexistence in a decidedly unpeaceful place. Don't get me started on Twitter.

Harold Varmus

Medical Scientist

Why I Write

Some of my fellow scientists and physicians have been writers in the conventional sense—think of C.P. Snow or Somerset Maugham—and more have written memoirs about their storied careers. But less attention has been drawn to the seemingly mundane writing that is obligatory for any investigator who wants to tell colleagues and the public about discoveries—both those achieved and those anticipated. My goal here is to say something about why we do that and its under-appreciated pleasures.

First, a few shards of relevant autobiography. My entry into science was atypical and involved transit through literary landscapes. I was born to health professionals whose parents were all immigrants from Eastern Europe. From my earliest days, I was an avid reader, but one who expected to practice medicine, not become a writer. After entering Amherst College, I found that I preferred seventeenth-century English poetry and editing the school newspaper to my pre-medical courses. So I went to graduate school, intending to get a PhD in British literature. But, once there, reading the greats and appraising them full-time, I got cold feet and retreated to medical school at Columbia University.

I was among the few who thoroughly enjoyed medical school—the human biology, the immersion in New York's urban culture, my first exposures to patients. But our country's military engagement in Vietnam obliged the most recent male graduates of American medical schools to serve in a war that I did not condone. So I sought and (surprisingly, with my limited laboratory experience) secured an exemption that allowed me to serve my time in a federal laboratory, at the National Institutes of Health (NIH), as part of the U.S. Public Health Service.

My scientific work went well, despite my history. Because I had quickly obtained experimental results that deserved to be told to others, it didn't take long to learn that writing was part of the deal. I remember with surprising clarity the moment over fifty years ago when my mentor

DOI: 10.4324/9781003516118-48

at the NIH said it was time to "write up" the first phase of my work for the esteemed *Journal of Biological Chemistry*.

The task seemed relatively simple compared to a graduate school essay about a Donne elegy or my undergraduate thesis on Charles Dickens. But it was more complex than what I had imagined to be the main compositional challenge for a scientist: keeping an accurate account of daily experimental work in a lab notebook. Still, the pages awaiting me were not blank sheets, as in my English courses. I was expected to conform to a traditional template for an article in a science journal—with a title and abstract, followed by crisply defined sections with their expected contents and style: the Introduction, Methods, Results, Discussion and References.

Further, much of the task required descriptions of many things that lacked ambiguity—from the contents of solutions (in Methods) to the design of experiments and the machine-rendered numerical outcomes of experiments (in Results). So it was not hard to type out a draft, formulate some figures and tables and taste one of the pleasures of scientific writing: praise—in this case, from my co-workers and other colleagues, for the speed and clarity of my composition.

Still, something was missing from the early draft. The account was dry. It had chronological fidelity but no narrative drive. It didn't fully explain why I had performed the experiments or what they might mean, and it didn't excite readers about what might be done next to extend the story to a new level of understanding.

When sent by the journal to members of its editorial board for peer review—by people who were much more mature than my actual peers at that stage—I was delighted to receive engaged responses that suggested how I could make the account into a story: How I could re-order the descriptions, even if the sequence of events did not conform to the order in which experiments were actually done. How I might engage readers and illuminate the significance of the story by making it more logical, even more suspenseful—without, of course, taking any liberties with the experimental findings themselves.

It did not take long to realize that writing in this way was not simply a chore. It offered a chance to organize my thoughts and my work in a way that told a tale that others enjoyed and remembered. It was also a way for me to better understand the importance and limits of my work, and to speculate about how it could be extended further and perhaps understood more profoundly.

Even at this early stage of learning to write about my laboratory work, I was receiving the stimuli that keep scientists engaged: the sensation that others might be interested in—even fascinated by or respectful of—the results. The bacterial geneticist and provocative essayist, Gunther Stent, speculated that he would be unlikely to do scientific work on a desert island if there were no one he could tell about his findings. Francis Crick, one half of the pair who discovered the helical pairing of DNA strands, gauged his own interest in scientific problems by what he called "the gossip factor"—whether he enjoyed telling someone else about a problem he was mulling over.

At this point, I realized how much I was coming to love experimental work because I was excited by its potential for discovering things that were entirely new and for answering questions that were previously unanswered or even previously asked. That was happening in part because I liked describing how discovery happened and getting praised by readers for doing so. The outcome was career-changing and dramatic: I abandoned clinical medicine to undertake laboratory work full-time.

But—as I also learned in those early days and have had repeatedly reinforced thereafter—scientists generally write because they must, not just because they sometimes enjoy the product. It is an inherent imperative: work that is done but not reported is no better in the long run than work that has not been done. Moreover, if a scientist wishes to do independent work but does not write, there will be no career, no jobs, no grants, and certainly no patents or prizes. There will be none of the status and gratification that go with the term "principal investigator."

There are, of course, other ways to be a scientist and contribute to science: by supporting the work of other individuals, of teams or of institutions, leaving the writing—and the design, conduct and interpretation of experiments—to others. But scientific reports that recount observations and experiments can reveal how discovery occurs, and how some portion of the universe, even a very small one, has been illuminated by hard work. In this sense, the act of writing a scientific report is an essential feature at the heart of science, as well as a source of pleasure for those who carry it out. Ultimately it is like all writing: an attempt to reveal what human beings have learned about their world and how that learning occurred.

Reference List

Editors' Introduction

Cather, Willa. *On Writing*. Knopf, 1949.

Freud, Sigmund. *Beyond the Pleasure Principle*. International Psycho-Analytical Press, 1920.

Freud, Sigmund. "Creative Writers and Day-Dreaming." Standard Edition, 9:141–154, Hogarth Press. 1908.

Orwell, George. "Why I Write." *Gangrel*, 1946.

Chapter 1 Models and Mentors

Babel, Isaac. *The Collected Stories of Isaac Babel*. Translated by Walter Morison, Plume, 1974.

Baldwin, James. *The Fire Next Time*. Vintage International, 1993.

Carroll, Lewis. *Through the Looking-Glass*. Macmillan, 1872.

Convery, Stephanie. "Terry Pratchett's Unfinished Novels Destroyed by Steamroller." *The Guardian*, 2017.

de Biasi, Pierre-Marc. "What Is a Literary Draft?" École Normale Supérieure, February 1995.

Dickens, Charles. *A Tale of Two Cities*. James Nisbet & Company, Ltd., 1902.

Didion, Joan. *The White Album*. Simon & Schuster, 1979.

Didion, Joan. "Why I Write." *The New York Times Book Review*, 1976.

Didion, Joan. *The Year of Magical Thinking*. Alfred A. Knopf, 2005.

Douglass, Frederick. "What to the Slave Is the Fourth of July?" Oration Delivered in Corinthian Hall, Rochester, 5 July 1852.

Ellison, Ralph. *Three Days Before the Shooting . . . .* Random House, 2011.

King, Jr., Martin Luther. "Letter from Birmingham Jail." 1963.

Lamb, Charles. *Essays of Elia*. Edward Moxon, 1833.

Miller, D.A. *Jane Austen, or the Secret of Style*. Princeton UP, 2005.

Orwell, George. "Why I Write." *Gangrel*, 1946.

Pegeen Kelly, Brigit. *Song*. BOA Editions, Ltd., 1995.

Poe, Edgar Allan. "The Importance of the Single Effect in a Prose Tale." The Poetry Foundation, 2009.

Stoute, Beverly. "Black Rage: The Psychic Adaptation to the Trauma of Oppression." *Journal of the American Psychoanalytic Association*, vol. 69, no. 2, 2021, pp. 259–90.

Stoute, Beverly. "Is Rage the Mitigating Force That Saves Us?" Plenary Panel Presentation at the Virtual Meeting of the American Psychoanalytic Association, 19 June 2020.

Stoute, Beverly. "The Racialized Mind Across the Life Cycle: Psychoanalytic Perspectives, the Michigan Psychoanalytic Society 47th Annual Symposium." The Saint Regis Hotel, Detroit, MI, 20 April 2024.

Whittemore, Amie. "Remembering Brigit Pegeen Kelly." *Amie Whittemore Blog*, 2016.

Williams, William Carlos. *Collected Poems: 1909–1939*. Vol. 1, New Directions, 1938.

Chapter 2 Urges and Traumas

Blake, William. *The Poetical Works of William Blake*. Forgotten Books, 2018.

Boyers, Peg. "An Interview with Natalia Ginzburg." *Salmagundi*, vol. 96, 1992.

Buber, Martin. *I and Thou*. Charles Scribner's Sons, 1923.

Chodorow, Nancy J. *The Reproduction of Mothering*. U of California P, 1978.

Cioran, E.M. *The Temptation to Exist*. U of Chicago P, 1998.

Didion, Joan. *Slouching Toward Bethlehem*. Farrar, Straus and Giroux, 1968.

Eliot, T.S. *Collected Poems, 1909–1962*. HarperCollins (Ecco), 2022.

Erikson, Erik. *Childhood and Society*. W.W. Norton & Co., 1950.

Glück, Louise. *Marigold and Rose: A Fiction*. Farrar, Straus and Giroux, 2022.

Keats, John. "Ode on a Grecian Urn." *Annals of the Fine Arts*, 1819.

Keats, John. "Ode to a Nightingale." *Annals of the Fine Arts*, 1819.

Martin, Marilyn. *Saving Our Last Nerve*. Hilton Publishing, 2002.

McGarry, Jean. *Airs of Providence*. Johns Hopkins UP, 2000.

McGarry, Jean. *Ocean State*. Johns Hopkins UP, 2010.

McGarry, Jean. *The Very Rich Hours*. Johns Hopkins UP, 1987.

O'Neill, Eugene. *Long Day's Journey into Night*. Yale UP, 2014.

Phillips, Carl. *In the Blood*. Northeastern UP, 1992.

Rolland, Romain. *The Enchanted Soul*. Albin Michel, 1923.

Rolland, Romain. *Jean-Christophe*. Modern Library, 1910.

Rolland, Romain. *Letters to Joseph Stalin (1935–1937)*. Translated by Paresh Chattopadhyay, Frontier, 2016.

Schultz, Philip. *Failure*. Ecco, 2009.

Slevin, Michael. "Of Being and Becoming: Psychoanalysis, Race and Class in an Urban ER." *The Psychoanalytic Study of the Child*, vol. 74, no. 1, 2021, pp. 77–89.

Whitman, Walt. *Leaves of Grass*. Self-Published, 1855.

Yeats, W.B. *The Collected Poems of W. B. Yeats*. Scribner, 1996.

Chapter 3 Evidence and Experiences

Baldwin, James. "Blacks and Jews." *The Black Scholar*, vol. 19, no. 6, 1988, pp. 3–15.

Bloom, James D. *The Stock of Available Reality: R.P. Blackmur and John Berryman*. UNKNO, 1985.

Dickens, Charles. *A Tale of Two Cities*. 1859. Bantam Books, 1981.

Eliot, T.S. *Collected Poems, 1909–1962*. HarperCollins (Ecco), 2022.

Flaubert, Gustave, and Eleanor Marx Aveling. *Madame Bovary*. A.A. Knopf, 1919.

Forster, E.M. *Aspects of the Novel*. Edward Arnold, 1927.

Frazier, Ian. *Great Plains*. Picador, 2001.

Freud, Sigmund. *Beyond the Pleasure Principle*. International Psycho-Analytical Press, 1920.

Freud, Sigmund. "Formulations on the Two Principles of Mental Functioning." Standard Edition, 12:213–226, Hogarth Press. 1911.

Hartley, Marsden. *Somehow a Past*. MIT Press, 1998.

Kafka, Franz. "A Hunger Artist." *Die neue Rundschau*, 1922.

Locke, John. *Second Treatise of Government*. Edited by C. B. Macpherson, Hackett Publishing Company, 1980.

Lopate, Phillip. *The Golden Age of the American Essay*. Anchor, 2021.

Marias, Javier. *When I Was Mortal*. New Directions, 2000.

Mitchell, Margaret. *Gone with the Wind*. Macmillan, 1936.

Obama, Barack. "Speech at the 2008 Iowa Caucus." Iowa Caucus, Iowa Democratic Party, 3 January 2008.

O'Keeffe, Georgia. "From the Faraway, Nearby." 1937, Oil on Canvas.

Orwell, George. "Why I Write." *Gangrel*, 1946.

Pascal, Blaise. *Lettres Provinciales*, 1857.

Shakespeare, William. *Hamlet*. Edited by George Richard Hibbard. Oxford UP, 2008.

Simon & Garfunkel. "Bridge Over Troubled Water." Columbia Records, 1969.

"Will Rogers—Even If You're on the Right Track, You'll..." *Brainyquote*, www.brainyquote.com/quotes/will_rogers_104938.

Index

Page numbers in *italics* indicate figures.

9781032850115